FIRST AID MANUAL

Editor
C. Savona-Ventura

Malta
2021

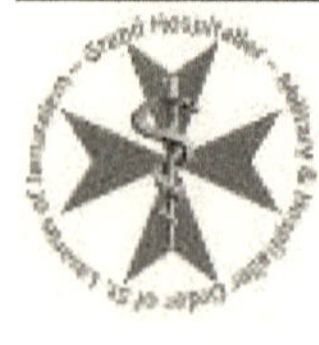

First Aid Manual
© Grand Priory of the Maltese Islands - MHOSLJ, Malta, 2021
Publisher: Lulu.com
ISBN: 978-1-7947-4683-1

Contents

What is a First Aider? 5

Psychological aspects of First Aid provision.............................13

The Emergency First Aid Kit 17

First Response: CPR and using an Automated External Defibrillator.......23

Controlling bleeding and treating shock 39

Managing the airway and treating choking [Heimlich manoeuvre] 39

Managing soft tissue injuries and burns 59

Managing skeletal injuries including fractures and potential spinal injuries 69

Management of poisoning 85

Animal bites or stings...93

Allergy and Anaphylaxis 101

Medical Emergencies 103

Obstetric Emergencies 121

Paediatric Emergencies 127

Emergency Numbers...143

Contributors 151

What is a First Aider?

Introduction

First aid is the administration of the immediate assistance given to any person suffering from illness or injury. It aims to provide care to preserve life, to prevent the condition from worsening, and/or to promote recovery. The First Aider aims to provide the essential initial intervention in situations where medical care is required prior to the availability of professional medical help. This assistance may involve providing treatment for injuries such as controlling blood loss in cases of trauma or performing cardiopulmonary resuscitation (CPR) while waiting for medical assistance.

The First Aider would ideally be someone with basic medical training in the principles of providing emergency aid or treatment given to someone who is injured, or falls suddenly ill, etc., before regular medical services arrive or can be reached. However, in the absence of trained personnel, anybody with basic knowledge of the concepts of first aid delivery can save lives. First aid very often involves making common sense decisions in the best interest of an injured or ill person. It is important to emphasize that first aid provision is not the provision of medical treatment and in no way can first aid be compared with what a trained medical professional can provide.

The primary goal of first aid is to provide help to prevent death or prevent serious injury from worsening. The key aims of first aid can be summarized with the acronym of 'the three Ps':

- *Preserve life*: The overriding aim of first aid is to save lives and minimize the threat of death.

- *Prevent further harm*: Measures should be instituted to prevent further harm or deterioration from developing. These measures may include simply ensuring a safe environment for the patient, e.g., removing the source of the harm, or apply first aid measures to prevent worsening of the condition, e.g., applying pressure to stop bleeding. Ideally an injured person should not be moved.

- *Promote recovery*: The First Aid assistance itself might also include measures that contribute to the recovery process from the illness or injury involving an integral step in the treatment regimen.

The need to provide first aid can arise at any time and in any circumstance. It may become necessary in situations where specific equipment may be available, e.g., in the workplace, or in situations where first aid equipment is completely unavailable requiring improvisation with materials available at the time. The first witness of an accident plays an essential role in the survival chain, and therefore the public should be encouraged to learn first aid since they are often the first who are present on the spot and thus can serve as a vital first link in the pre-hospital care. The more people that are trained in First Aid provision, the more the community benefits.

Qualities of a First Aider

Anybody may find him/herself in a position where first aid needs to be provided. This intervention, when done effectively and efficiently, can help save lives. The First Aider should ideally have developed specific qualities for effective management.

- *Skilled & resourceful*: The First Aider should be skilled in basic first aid techniques, and thus be able to judge the situation and institute the right management with confidence. This of course is very much dependent on the level of training one has undergone.

The more advanced the training, the higher the level of skill and confidence. The First Aider needs to be resourceful and look for alternative equipment is the standard required materials are unavailable.

- *Quick & decisive*: First aid providers must be very quick in their response and take control over the situation without any delay. It is often essential that a quick decision is made as to the course of action that needs to be taken in the circumstances. Hesitation will contribute to the generation of panic compounding the situation. The First Aider needs to assume the role of leader in the situation and, if necessary, garner help from the crowd.

- *Controlled & reassuring*: The person providing first aid must show confidence in the measures being undertaken. The situation in hand very often will be one where a sense of panic prevails in the victim and in those around. By showing confidence in the actions taken, the First Aider will help maintain a controlled and calm environment. At the same time, First Aid providers need to repeatedly reassure the victim and the onlookers that everything is in hand and under control.

- *Team player*: Teamwork and communication is essential in emergency situations. The First Aider needs to work and communicate effectively with the people around, with other first aiders, and with medical staff. Effectively delivered messages can ensure public safety and facilitate response efforts.

Responsibilities of a First Aider

The first aider is to provide immediate, potentially lifesaving, medical care, before the arrival of further medical help. Anyone assuming the role of a lead first aider in an emergency needs to apply the basic principles of First Aid before undertaking to manage the incident. The basic principles of First Aid is to meet the immediate needs of the casualty who may be seriously sick or injured, before formal medical aid is available and to prevent the condition from worsening.

A. Ensure the continuing safety of him/herself, any bystanders, and the victim. Manage bystanders effectively with good crowd control.

B. Assess the nature & extent of the injury or illness and monitor vital signs. Find out if the casualty's pulse is beating and whether he/she is breathing regularly → if the pulse and/or breathing are absent, then check that the airway is clear and start cardiorespiratory resuscitation immediately.

C. Arrange for further medical help or other emergency services to be called in all situations of serious illness or injury especially in the presence of broken bones or severe bleeding.

D. Reassure while keeping the victim at rest until help arrives.

E. Provide appropriate and reasonable first aid management depending on the circumstances.

- If the casualty is conscious, ask for details of what happened and if he/she is in pain. This will help you decide on the extent of the injury or the type of illness you may be dealing with.
- If the casualty is unconscious, then place in the recovery position → turn him/her onto the uninjured side with the arm of this side behind the back; bend the knee of this side slightly. Place the other arm in a convenient position, bring both the hip and knee on this side to almost a right-angle. Be careful in situations where you suspect a spinal or neck injury.

- If bleeding, control the bleeding by direct pressure on the bleeding site.

F. Provide a handover summary of circumstances and management given when further medical help arrives.

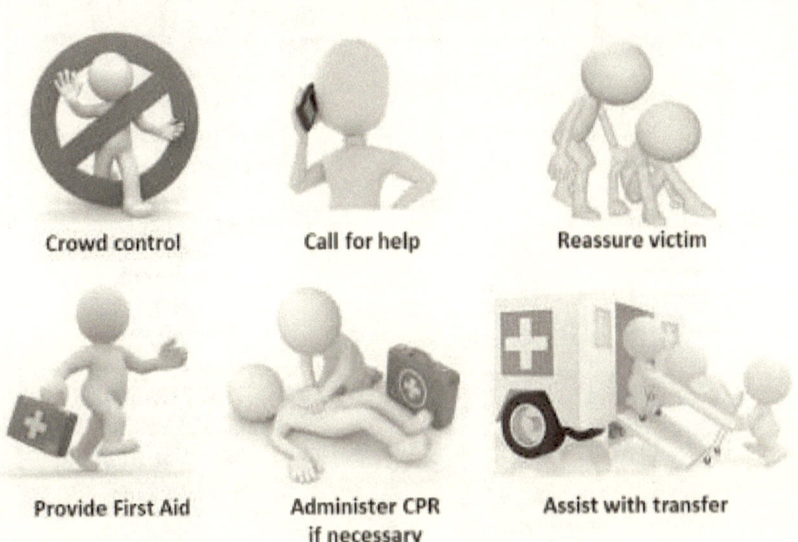

EMERGENCY MANAGEMENT

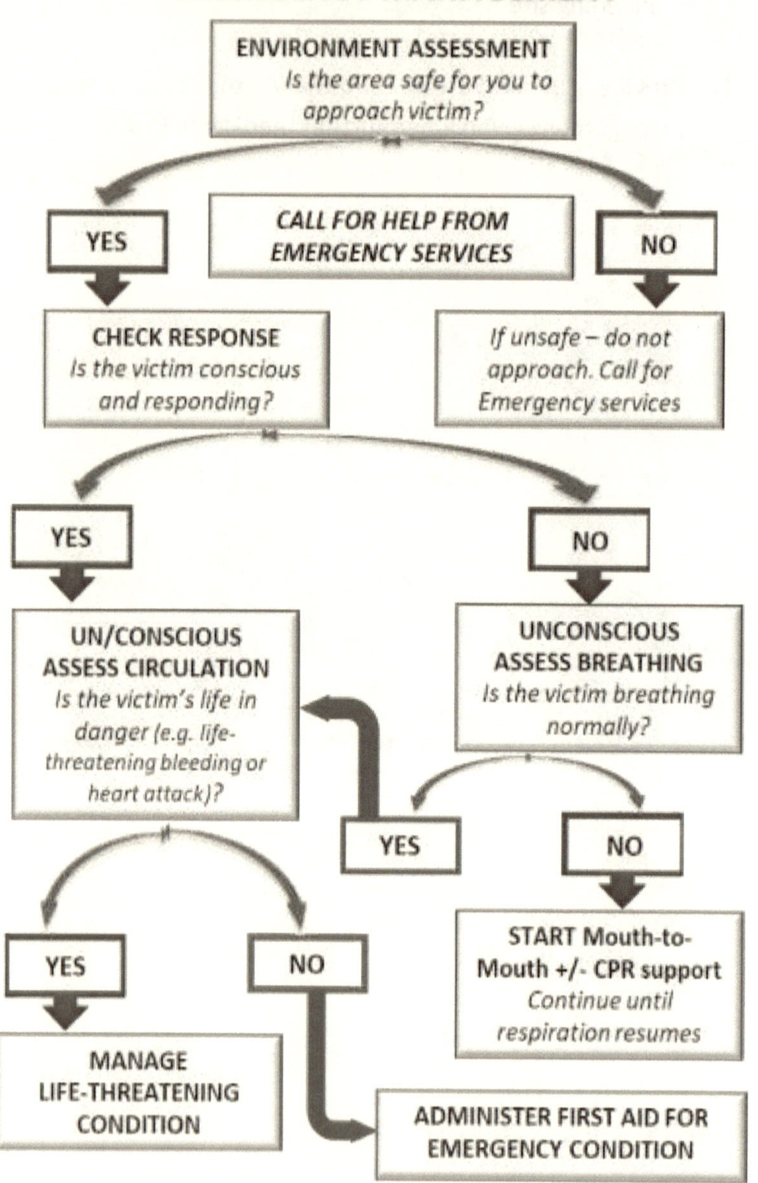

Essential life-saving skills

Essential first aid skills that everyone should become familiar with include:

- *The Heimlich manoeuvre.* This is a first aid procedure used to treat upper airway obstructions (or choking) by foreign objects.

- *Stopping heavy bleeding.* Continuous bleeding will contribute towards hypovolaemia causing the body to shut down. The first stage of hypovolaemic shock occurs when about 15% of the total blood volume (equivalent to about 750 ml) is lost.

- *Treating shock.* Shock can result from haemorrhage or severe pain response. It is important for the First Aider to identify the aetiology and manage appropriately.

- *Hypothermia treatment.* Hypothermia occurs when body heat is lost faster that it is generated. This generally occurs in situations where the victim is exposed to cold-weather conditions or cold water. Appropriate first aid measure can help save the victim's like.

- *Using an Automatic External Defibrillator (AED).* Most establishments have introduced an AED station to help first aiders assist individuals suffering a heart attack. It is therefore essential that First Aiders are familiar with the use of this equipment.

- *Knowing the signs of a stroke.* Timely medical intervention of stroke may reduce the consequence of the vent. It is therefore essential for a First Aider to identify the early signs of stroke.

Multiple victim situation - triage

The First Aider may be faced with a multiple victim situation where assistance may be needed by more than one individual. In such situations it is important to recruit the assistance of others who may be present on the scene. Teamwork and collaboration are essential to ensure maximal delivery of effective emergency services and needs to all the victims.

However, the First Aider must get stock of the situation and triage the victims as to the severity of the injuries and the urgency needed to deal with these. The formal triage chart classifies victims into five categories.

RED	*Immediate*	Victims with life-threatening injuries that are treatable with a minimum amount of time and supplies. Good chance of recovery.
YELLOW	*Urgent*	Victims whose treatment may be delayed for a limited period of time without incurring significant adverse consequences.
GREEN	*Delayed*	Victims with minor injuries whose treatment may be delayed indefinitely without consequences until more urgent victims are dealt with.
BLUE	*Expectant*	Victims whose injuries are so extensive that are beyond the limited aid available in the circumstances.
BLACK	*Dead*	Victims that show no signs of life.

Psychological aspects of First Aid provision

Introduction

In all emergency situations, the provision of first aid and the calling of assistance from rescue services is the top priority in first aid management. However, the psychological support for the injured and other involved people in the emergency event is no less important. It is important that until the rescue services arrive, the First Aider must provide a feeling of security in a calming and understanding manner to all those involved in the incident. Fear, panic, helplessness, and aggressiveness can develop very quickly in the absence of suitable support.

One needs not be a professional psychologist to help someone in need. What is needed is committed action, empathy, and compassion. It must be remembered that individuals may show different psychological behaviours when faced with unusual situations such as emergencies. For example, some individuals may react helplessly and fearfully, while others in the same situation may panic or become aggressive. Psychological support may need to be provided not only injured or sick individuals, but also to other participants in the situation such as those who caused the accident, relatives, bystanders, or helpers. It is important to let the persons concerned know that their psychological reactions are normal and that, with their reaction, they are helping to process their experience.

The victim may experience a panic attack resulting in hyperventilation causing light-headedness and a feeling of tingling in the fingers as well as around the mouth [see *Medical Emergencies* below]

The 4-core rule for psychological first aid

The 4-core rule serves as a useful guideline framework for providing psychological care to emergency patients. The principles of the rule involve:

- REASSURANCE: When handling an emergency, it is important to explain that someone is there and that something is happening.

Say that you are there, and that help is coming or is there.

Those affected by the circumstances should feel that they are not alone. Even simply stating: "I'll stay with you until the ambulance comes" may have a relieving and calming effect. The victims should also be informed about intended and already implemented measures, such as "The ambulance is on the way".

- COMMUNICATION: Talking to the victims can be beneficial to help establish a

Speak and listen actively with the victims

good line of communication and develop reassurance. Introduce yourself by name and ask for the victim's name. Listen patiently when people talk and make eye contact. Try not to transmit a sense of panic by becoming hectic and adjust your conversation volume to the circumstances. You can also ask the person questions to keep the conversation going. If the person has lost consciousness, continue to speak to them in a calm voice anyway.

- PHYSICAL CONTACT: Many victims find light body contact pleasant and calming.

Slowly seek physical contact with the victim.

Therefore, hold the hand or shoulder of the person concerned. Touching the head or other parts of the body, however, is not recommended. Stand at the same height as those affected, preferably kneeling next to them.

If people are constrained by clothing or the cold, remedy this by opening a few buttons or covering them with something to keep them warm.

- SHIELD: Inquisitive looks are uncomfortable for the victims. Discourage onlookers in a

> *Shield the victim from onlookers.*

friendly but firm manner by saying: "Stand back, we need space." If viewers are annoying because they give unnecessary advice or tell of their own experiences, it may be useful to assign them tasks. For example, an onlooker's help can be recruited to secure the scene of the accident or to keep other onlookers at a distance.

Always try to speak in a calm voice and stay calm with any remarks against you or others present! One must
at all costs avoid making comments about the incident. Thus, one should:
- Avoid all forms of criticism or accusations such as: "You were traveling too fast" or "You drank way too much!"
- Avoid any comment or speculation on the question of guilt.
- Hold back your opinion and try not to force a problem solution.
- Do not provide details about the extent of the event or the number of people affected.
- Do not speculate about the type and severity of injuries.
- Do not provide any information about any dead victims or possibly danger-of-dying victims.

The Emergency First Aid Kit

Introduction

Almost everyone will be faced with an emergency in the home or in the community at some time or another. It is important to be prepared as much as possible for all possible common eventualities. This includes the availability of a First Aid kit in the home and preferably in the car. First aid kits may be basic or comprehensive, depending on the extent of your First Aid capabilities. However, it is always better to be over-prepared rather than underprepared. Ready-made first aid kits are commercially available from chain stores or outdoor retailers. But you can make a simple and inexpensive first aid kit yourself. Remember that that any included medications have an expiry date, so it is important to occasionally review and replace any expired or due-to-expire items in the kit.

Contents

Home first aid kits are usually used for treating minor traumatic injuries such as burns, cuts and abrasions, insect strings, splinters, and sprains and strains. It should also include any medications that may be needed to counter the effects of specific medical conditions anyone in the family may suffer from – e.g., glucagon injection for diabetics on insulin, an epinephrine injection [EpiPen] for allergies, etc. Of course, a First Aid Manual can be included for easy reference.

Essential items in a first aid kit should include:

- Disposable sterile examination gloves
- Alcohol wipes

- Antiseptic agent (small bottle liquid soap) - for cleaning wounds and hands. A good alternative are packets of cleansing non-alcohol based wipes.
- Adhesive tape and Band-aid strips (various sizes)
- Safety pins (large and small)
- Small, medium, and large sterile gauze dressings
- Non-adhesive wound pads
- Moleskin - to apply to blisters.
- Rolled Bandages (all sizes ideally crepe bandages) and a triangular bandage
- Cigarette lighter - to sterilize instruments.
- Small flashlight
- Knife (small Swiss Army-type)
- Scissors
- Tweezers
- Thermometer (preferably digital)
- Plastic resealable bags (oven and sandwich)
- Pocket mask for CPR
- Emergency space thermal blanket
- Instant cold pack
- Eye wash cup and sterile eye pads
- Antibiotic ointment
- Antihistamine cream
- An oral antihistamine (e.g., Diphenhydramine)
- Corticosteroid cream
- Pain killers – aspirin / paracetamol / ibuprofen

First aid kits for travel need to be more comprehensive and would ideally also include medications for minor disturbing symptomatology such as indigestion, diarrhoea, congested nose, and cough. When travelling in a hot country, rehydration sachets are essential components especially if travelling with young children. Make sure that a sunscreen cream of at least an SPF value of 30-50 is available. It is furthermore important that you ensure that facilities to contact emergency services. Including a phonecard with at least 60 minute talking time may be a useful addition – mobile phones are only useful if they are charged and functional. When travelling, remember also to include a sufficient stock of any personal medications with perhaps some extra. These are best carried as hand luggage to ensure timely arrival. A travel medical kit would therefore include:

- Rehydration sachets
- 30-50 SPF sunscreen cream
- Insect repellent
- Antiacid preparation
- Antidiarrheal agent [e.g., Imodium]
- Cough medication
- Nasal spray and oral decongestant

Further useful items to be included in a First Aid kit

Airways: An oropharyngeal airway, e.g. Gujedel airway, is a useful tool to have available to ensure that the airway remains clear. Its design ensures that the victim's tongue does not fall back and block the airway. This is particularly useful in those situations when the victim's condition requires him/her to be on the back, e.g. to apply cardiopulmonary resuscitation or in suspected spinal injuries when the victim cannot be placed in the recovery position. Before use, inspect the victim's airway; insert the airway to a third of its length with the end pointing to the roof of the mouth, then turn it through 180^0 to point down to the throat. Various colour-coded sizes are available – ideally have at least two suitable to use in adults and children – usually the black (Size no. 1, length 60 mm suitable for a child) and the green (Size no. 3, length 80 mm suitable for an adult) will suffice.

Size		Length	Colour code
00	Neonatal	40 mm	Pink
0	Infant	50 mm	Light blue
1	Child	60 mm	Black
2	Small adult	70 mm	White
3	Adult	80 mm	Green
4	Large adult	90 mm	Yellow
5	XL adult	100 mm	Red
6	XXL adult	110 mm	Orange

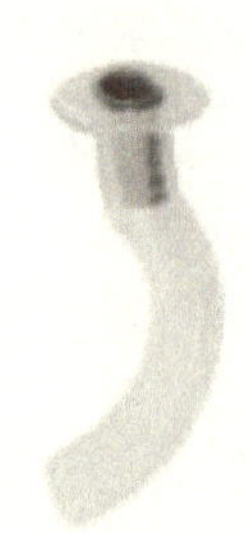

Gujedel oropharyngeal airways chart

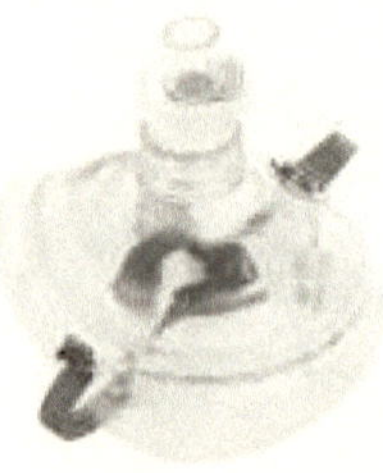

A CPR pocket mask to assist with mouth-to-mouth resuscitation is another useful item to include in a professional first aid kit. This ensures that a good seal is maintained over the nose and mouth and is particularly useful to prevent the transfer of any liquid or air containing potential pathogens to the First Aider.

A Mucus extractor to clear the airway from any fluids within the airway is another useful implement. This can be used directly through the victim's mouth or placed down the artificial airway. Its one-way valve allows the fluids to be sucked out without the risk of the First Aider swallowing this accidentally. If unavailable, one can use any tube or straw, but this does carry the risk of accidentally swallowing the fluid.

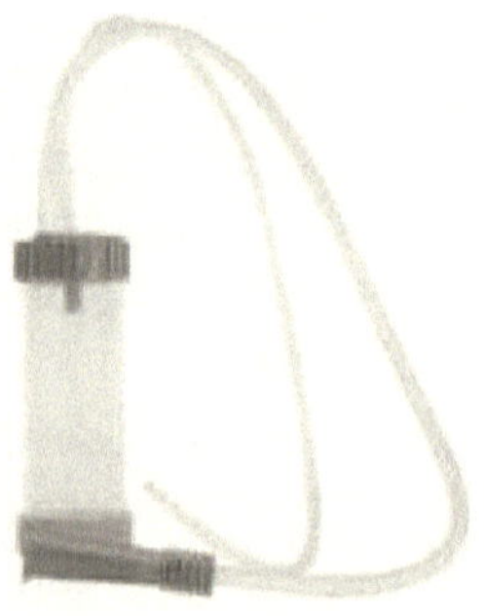

Bandages: The triangular or cravat bandage with short sides measuring about 1 meter is a very useful and versatile dressing. It can be used to serve as a sling or folded to make a wide range of supports and bandages. Roll bandages may be made of two varieties – open weave gauze or crepe material. The latter are easier to apply, apply pressure more evenly, and are less likely to come loose. The less bulky gauze bandages are useful for restricted areas where the rather bulky crepe material may hinder adequate bandaging, e.g. finger bandaging. Ideally, pack at least one triangular bandage, four roll crepe bandages, and one gauze bandage. When applying bandages, remember that that these should be applied firmly to avoid them slipping but NOT too tight to interfere with the circulation or cause discomfort. Check regularly the bandaged limb for a restricted circulation looking for any signs of blueness at the extremities.

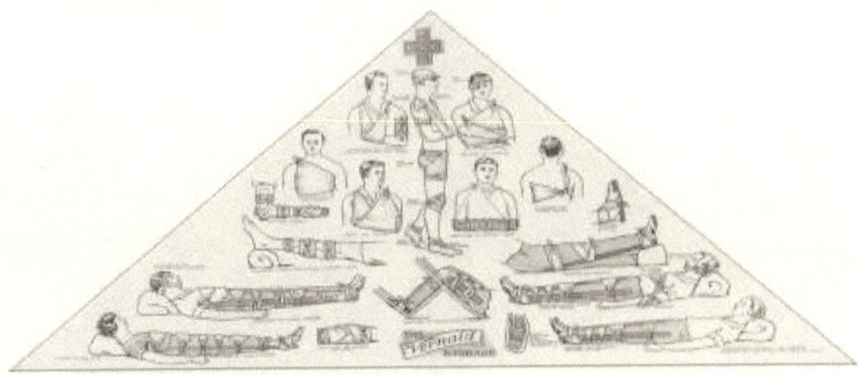

An early 20th century Vernaid triangular bandage with instructions

Dressings: These usually consist of a pad of cotton wool covered with gauze and attached to a bandage or an adhesive strip in a sterile wrapping. The dressing is applied to the wound without touching the dressing pad. Never use cotton wool directly on an open wound since this will adhere to the surface. In an emergency, one can improvise suitable dressings from any clean material available. Try to include at least two 4" x 4" sterile gauze pad dressing in your First Aid kit.

Antiseptic: An antiseptic is a substance that stops or slows down bacterial growth. It should be used to wash one's hands before managing open wounds. It is also useful when cleaning superficial skin injuries such as cuts and abrasions; however, antiseptics should not be applied to deep wounds since they may cause further tissue damage. Chlorhexidine or dilute betadine solution are standard all-purpose antiseptics, but a simple soap solution is also an excellent alternative. The antiseptic can be mixed with water, ideally preboiled. If this is unavailable, urine can be used. Urine is a sterile fluid and thus will not introduce infection. It also itself has a slight antiseptic function through the presence of uric acid.

First Response: CPR and using an Automated External Defibrillator

Introduction

Cardiac arrest occurs suddenly and often without any warning. Thousands die every year around the world and many lives can be saved if cardiac arrest is recognised early by responding bystanders who are close at hand and assist the victim in initiating early resuscitative efforts through effective cardiopulmonary resuscitation or CPR. These efforts will include high quality chest compressions with or without accompanying rescue breathing and possibly subsequent defibrillation through the use of an automated external defibrillator. These lifesaving machines are now frequently set up in strategic locations within the Community and thus are more easily accessible when required urgently. Cardiopulmonary resuscitation is also known as Basic Life Support / AED and can be successfully performed by bystanders having little or no prior training in life saving skills by simply following dispatcher-assisted telephone CPR instructions when calling the EMS emergency number of the Country. Having prior resuscitation experience through CPR courses is obviously a bonus.

Initiating Basic Life support early through high-quality chest compressions and rescue breaths will improve blood flow to a heart in cardiac arrest. As this has stopped pumping blood effectively, adequate oxygen transference to the brain is essential in view of increasing hypoxia due to the cardiac arrest state. Isolated CPR may not restart the heart, but it has been proven to prime the heart to respond positively to cardiac defibrillation through the use of an Automated External defibrillator (AED). Maintaining adequate circulation and oxygenation may offset major organ failure, mainly the heart and the brain, for a few essential minutes until defibrillation is carried out.

The following instructions are based on European Resuscitation Council (ERC) Guidelines 2021 aimed at initiating cardiopulmonary resuscitation in a victim who is in recognised cardiac arrest. Bystander CPR can double or even triple cardiac arrest survival so a little knowledge in CPR and a good pair of hands can go far in saving a life.

Chain of Survival

Only 8 – 10% of victims survive out of hospital cardiac arrest with a subsequent stable hospital discharge. These numbers strongly depend on sequential essential timely actions being carried out and these are aptly defined as the *Chain of Cardiac Arrest survival*. The first link in this tightly linked chain is early recognition of active cardiac arrest which triggers an call to activate the Emergency Response services (EMS) for urgent assistance. Early initiation of CPR with an emphasis on effective chest compressions in conjunction with early access to an Automated External Defibrillator (AED) and rapid defibrillation, significantly improves the chances of survival especially in those cases of cardiac collapse due to an irregular cardiac rhythm known as ventricular fibrillation (VF).

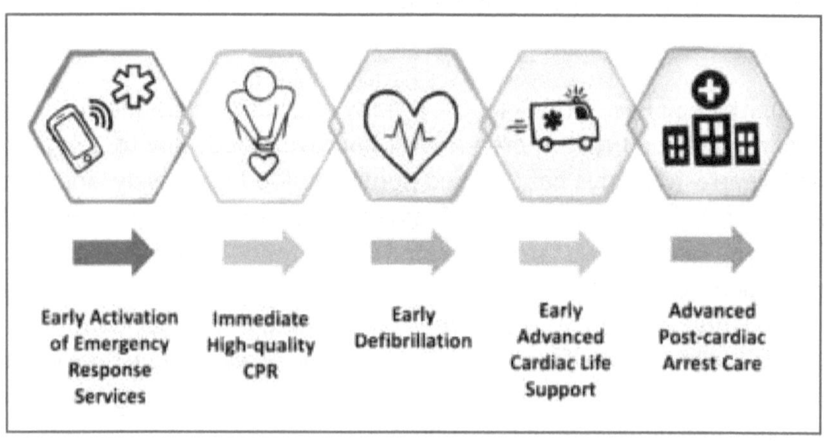

Initiating Basic life support plus early defibrillation within 3 to 5 minutes of collapse produces the highest survival rates. In fact, each minute of delayed Basic Life Support with defibrillation reduces the probability of survival to hospital discharge by 10% to 12%. The final links in the Chain of Survival are effective Advanced Life Support and in hospital post resuscitation management aimed at protecting cardiac and cerebral function. However, early recognition of cardiac arrest, activation of the EMS response and initiating CPR remain the greatest stumbling blocks to survival from cardiac arrest.

Recognising Cardiac Arrest

The first step in any emergency is the recognition of the problem and providing help. The ABCs of first aid are the primary things that need to be checked when you approach the victim, Airway, Breathing, and Circulation. Prior to CPR, ensure that the airway is clear, check to see if the patient is breathing, and check for circulation (pulse or observation of colour and temperature of hands/fingers).

> **Cardiac arrest is defined as having occurred if the victim is deemed unresponsiveness having associated absent or abnormal breathing.**

This should immediately trigger a response by bystanders to start the process of cardiopulmonary resuscitation. Thus, the presence of a person close having some basic training in first aid and life support skills remains the main limiting factor to optimal response towards a cardiac arrest scenario. The urgency of initiating lifesaving CPR is strongly emphasised ensuring early recognition that actual cardiac arrest has occurred in a witnessed victim collapse. Emergency system dispatchers can guide you through the steps of performing cardiopulmonary resuscitation (CPR), using an automatic external defibrillator (AED), or delivering basic care until additional help arrives.

It must be stressed that slow laboured breathing, also defined as *agonal breathing,* should be considered a sign of cardiac arrest. This abnormal breathing pattern occurs quite commonly and is often misinterpreted as regular breathing motion. This possibly delays the crucial onset of basic life support efforts in possibly decreasing subsequent survival.

In addition, actual recognition that cardiac arrest has occurred may be offset by *initial involuntary fits or seizures* in the victim which may occur early following collapse and thus confuse responding rescuers interpretation of the presenting symptoms.

Thus, in guidance, any persistence of unconsciousness associated with abnormal, or absent breathing or chest movements in the post fit period should automatically be interpreted as a cardiac arrest starting effective CPR.

Cardiac Arrest may be the result of multiple causes. This may be preceded by an episode of severe compressive chest pain indicating the onset of myocardial infarction or heart attack with associated abnormal cardiac rhythms. Asphyxia, choking, electrocution or drug overdose may be other causes. Whatever the aetiology for the cardiac arrest, safety of the responder is paramount and approach to scene of the collapsed victim should only be carried out if it is safe to do so.

1. Safe approach and initial assessment: Is the patient conscious?

The responder must approach the victim with care and attention to possible danger at scene, making sure that there is no further risk to self, the victim, or any other bystanders in the vicinity willing to assist. Look out especially for any live electrical cables, exposed wires or the possibility of gas being released within a closed environment. Always shout out for help and assistance from persons nearby.

- Call out to the victim and shake him gently by the shoulders and see if there is any visible response elicited.
- **If there is a visible positive response** to stimulation or calls then the victim should be left in the position found and the emergency medical services contacted, then getting back to the victim as quickly as possible to continue with any immediate needs.
- **If there is no visible positive response** to stimulation or calls, observe if the victim is breathing normally and is the chest rising and falling.

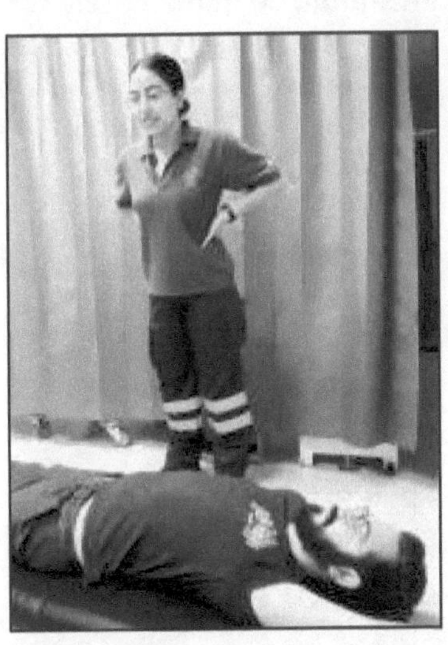
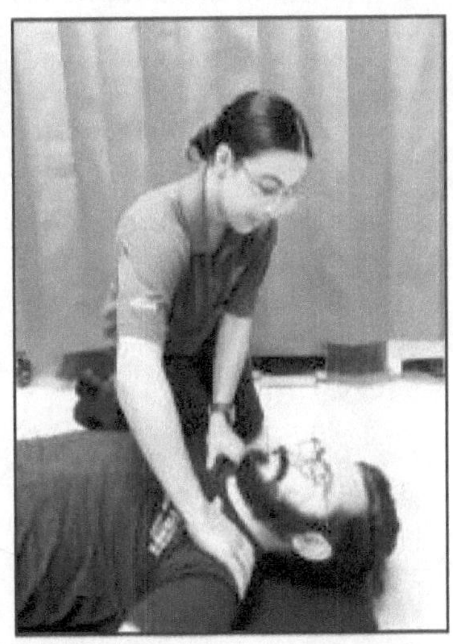

2. Safe approach and initial assessment: Is the patient breathing?

Absence of breathing may be due to the muscular tongue falling backwards and obstructing the airway. With the victim on his back, face up, initially tilt the head backwards by placing the palm of your hand on the patient's forehead and at the same time lifting the chin using two fingers under the chin. This may open the airway by pulling the tongue forwards. This action is termed the ***head tilt - chin lift manoeuvre*** and is easily carried out. This manoeuvre should not be carried out however if there is suspicion of trauma to the head or neck.

In checking to see if the patient is breathing and **LOOK * LISTEN * FEEL** for no more than 10 seconds. Look for the rise and fall of the chest seen in normal breathing movements. By placing your head close to the victim, look for chest movement, listen for breath sounds and feel for breathing movements on your cheek. If breathing is agonal in character, do not confuse this with normal breathing. If the breathing pattern is slow, laboured, or agonal in character then cardiac arrest should be assumed. **If no breathing is elicited in the unresponsive victim after 10 seconds of initial assessment, then CPR should be immediately started.**

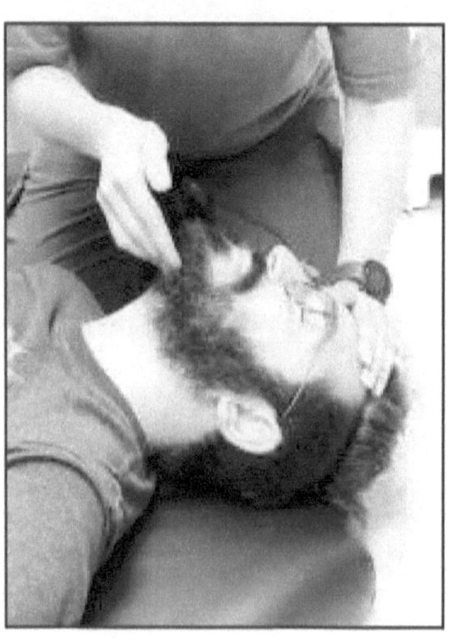
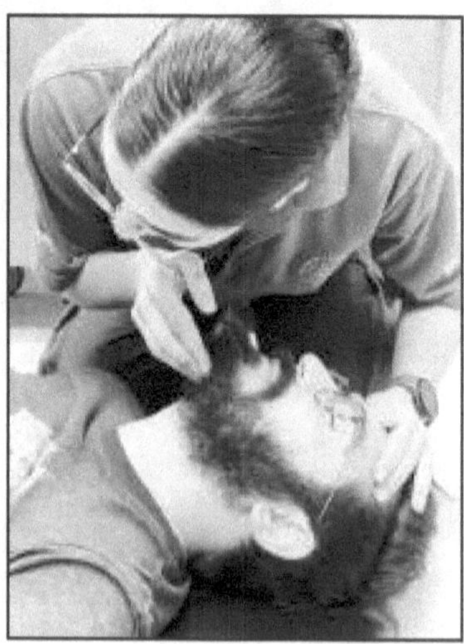

3. Alerting the Emergency Medical Services

With new mobile phone technology at hand, having one rescuer at scene, rather than two, should no longer delay starting CPR in informing the emergency medical services on the need of assistance to respond to a cardiac arrest incident. Through the handsfree loudspeaker function of a mobile phone the lone trained responder may place an emergency call to the EMS in passing on the necessary required information whilst initiating essential CPR. Even if the responder has little or no CPR training, the hands-free option of the mobile phone should be used to implement dispatcher assisted CPR.

Essential acceptable basic life support can thus be maintained through dispatcher assisted instructions on how to carry out continual chest compressions and even rescue breaths until the arrival of professional EMS services on scene to take over the CPR process.

If a mobile phone is not immediately at hand, it would be wise to prime the EMS services first and then promptly returning to the collapsed victim and initiating CPR.

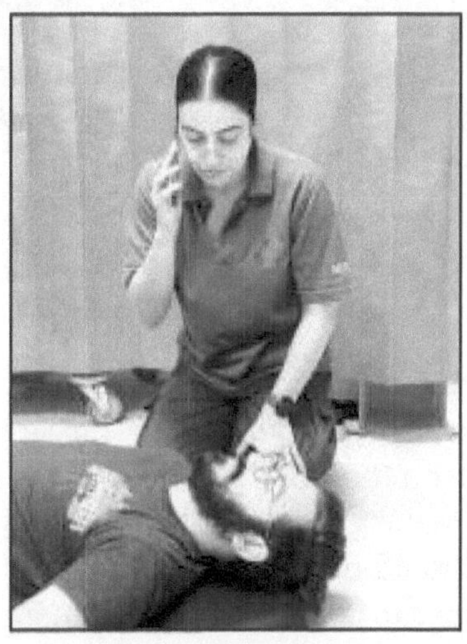

4. Initiate high quality chest compressions

Once cardiac arrest is recognised, it is imperative that all rescuers start chest compressions with minimum delay as possible. Ideally the patient should be placed supine on a firm hard surface to ensure maximum effectiveness of the chest compressions. If the collapse victim is lying on the floor, start by kneeling by his side and placing one hand over the other with fingers intertwined over the lower half of the sternum in the centre of the chest. This is done offset any unnecessary injuries to the ribs in compressing the chest wall during CPR.

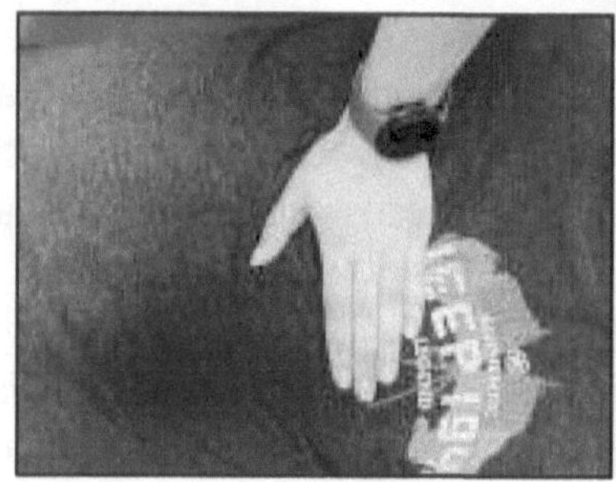 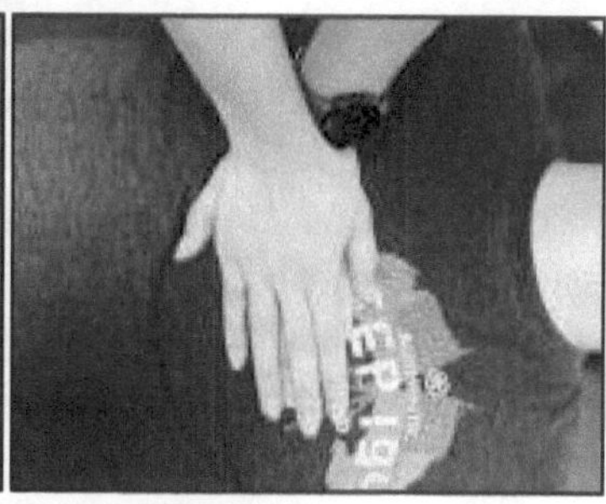

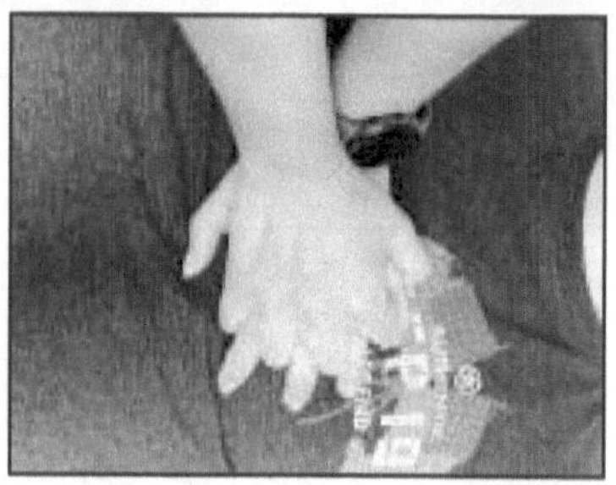

Chest compressions should be carried out at a rate of approximately 100 to 120 compressions per minute. Keep the arms and elbows straight whilst pushing hard on the chest to a depth of at least 5 cm. One should avoid any forward leaning movements in allowing full recoil of the chest wall. The hands should be kept in contact with the chest skin surface avoiding interruptions to compression movements.

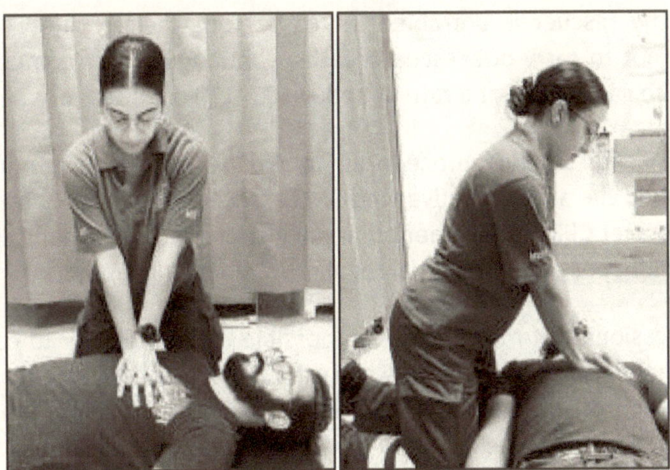

5. Rescue breaths

Trained emergency responders should be able to carry out combined chest compressions and rescue breaths. Two rescue breaths should be attempted following 30 high quality chest compressions.

Open the airway using the head tilt - chin lift manoeuvre whilst pinching the nose at the same time. After taking a good breath in, a good seal should be maintained by placing your lips around the victim's lips and blowing into the victim's mouth for about one second. A chest rise would ensure that proper ventilation is being carried out. This process is repeated for a second time. The time to deliver these two rescue breaths should not exceed ten seconds. Many protective shields and one-way valve breathing devices are available on the market to ensure increased responder safety in delivering rescue breaths.

If the chest does not rise following the rescue breath one should think about the possibility of an obstructed airway. Recheck the airway and reposition the head tilt chin left manoeuvre.

If the rescuer is untrained or for personal health safety reasons prefers not to carry out rescue breaths, continuous chest compressions should be carried out at a rate of about 100 -120 compressions a minute.

Basic life support procedures should be continued continuously either until the arrival of advanced EMS assistance on scene who in turn will take over CPR management or if the victim starts to respond showing signs of life, possibly with initial regular breathing movements.

Occasionally it may become impossible for the rescuer to continue CPR either because of sheer personal exhaustion being the sole responder on site or possibly because rescuer safety becomes compromised. In addition, a certified health care professional may decide to call for the cessation of additional CPR efforts due to the futility of further continual resuscitative measures.

6. Use of an Automated External Defibrillator (AED)

The widespread introduction of public access AEDs within the community has ensured that a lifesaving machine may be close at hand to the site of cardiac arrest. AEDs are simple, safe, and effective when used by either lay rescuers or health care professionals.

As soon as a defibrillator is made available, lift the lid, and follow the audible instructions given be the machine. Remove the electrodes pads and attach them to the victim's bare chest whilst removing clothing as is feasibly necessary. Although the electrode pads are interchangeable, diagrammatic advice on the electrode package will indicate the proper positioning of the pads. It is imperative that if there is more than one rescuer at scene, then chest compressions are continued by a second responder whilst the AED pads are being placed onto the chest.

The first pad should be placed just below the right clavicle or collarbone on the right anterior chest wall. The second electrode pad should be placed under the left armpit just laterally on the left anterior chest wall, ideally under the left breast in women.

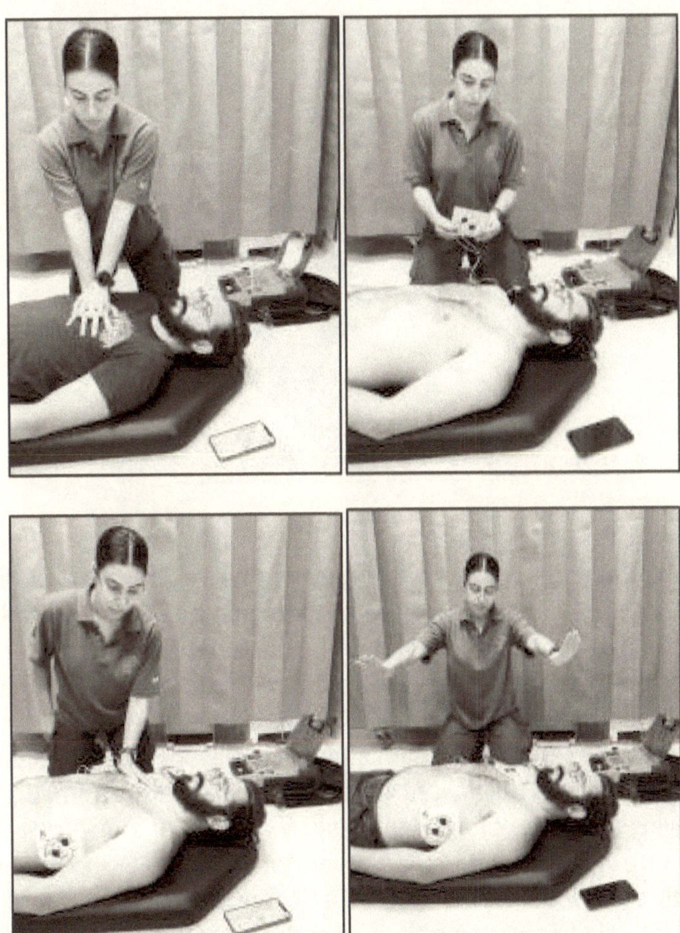

In placing the electrode pads on the chest, it is best to wipe the chest dry especially if the victim is wet consequent to a drowning incident or may be profusely sweaty due to an adverse cardiac event. Any visible plasters, jewellery, metal rings or medication patches should be removed prior to attempting defibrillation. The electrode pads should never be applied over possible cardiac pacemakers which are usually fitted subcutaneously just under the left collarbone.

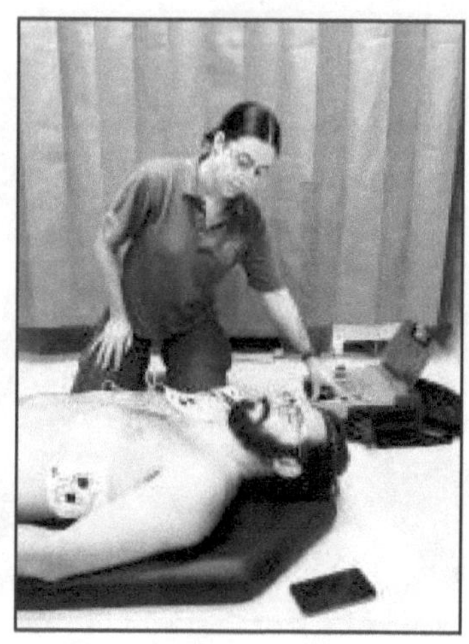

Whilst the AED analyses the presenting cardiac rhythm it is imperative that there is no movement to the victim's body during the process, as this will disrupt actual analysis and delay further actions. In preparation for possible defibrillation, the safety of the rescuers and other team members remains paramount and full safety measures taken during the handling of defibrillators and shock delivery. All other members of the responding team and any family members in the vicinity to the victim should be advised to 'stand back' from the immediate area in removing all danger of accidental injury passage of the electrical shock current to other responders. The operator of the AED should lead this advice through loud verbal and visual commands to stand back made understandable to all around the victim during resuscitation.

- ***If the victim is in a shockable rhythm***, the AED will indicate that a shock should be delivered advising the responder to push the flashing button on the AED. Alternatively, some AEDs can deliver an automated shock where the defibrillator will advise the responders to stand back whilst analysis of the presenting cardiac rhythm takes place and deliver a shock accordingly.

Interruption to the chest compression sequence period should be shortened with as minimum a delay as possible. Carrying out the rhythm analysis and possible shock sequence should take no longer than 10 seconds. Once the use of the AED is completed the 30 compressions to 2-rescue breath sequence should be restarted.

- ***If no shock is indicated*** by AED rhythm analysis the rescuer should continue with the resuscitation sequence process as is directed and prompted by the AED.

Ensure that EMS rescue services are on their way to scene, and CPR should be continued until professional assistance can take over. If cardiopulmonary resuscitation is successful with the victim showing signs of life by visibly breathing, demonstrating movement of the limbs, or actually regains consciousness, then all resuscitative processes should cease, and the victim should be placed in the ***Recovery Position***.

The Recovery Position

If a person is unconscious but is breathing and has no other life-threatening conditions, they should be placed in the recovery position. This will ensure that their airway remains open and clear without the risk of airway obstruction and choking from any possible vomit or food. There are 4 basic steps in placing the **unconscious but breathing victim** into the recovery position:

- **Step 1: Positioning the arms**:

With the patient on their back with their legs straight, kneel beside the patient and remove any spectacles and bulky or sharp objects in their pockets. Place the arm that is nearest to you at a right angle to their body, with the elbow bent and their palm facing upwards. Bring their other arm across their chest and place the back of their hand against the cheek nearest to you making sure it remains there.

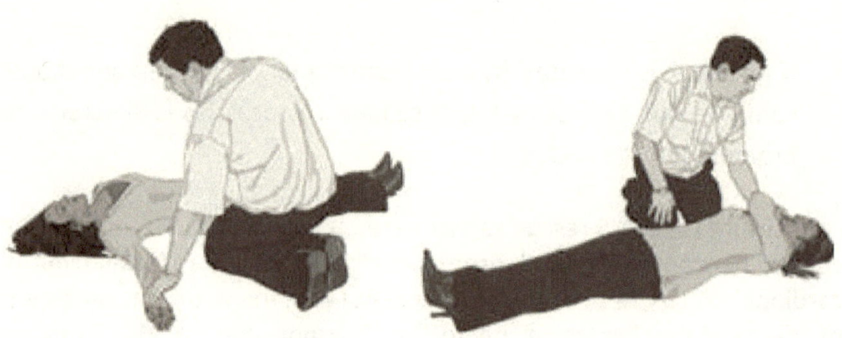

- **Step 2: Positioning the legs.**

With your other hand, pull the knee furthest away up so that their foot is flat on the floor.

- **Step 3: Rolling the patient into position.**

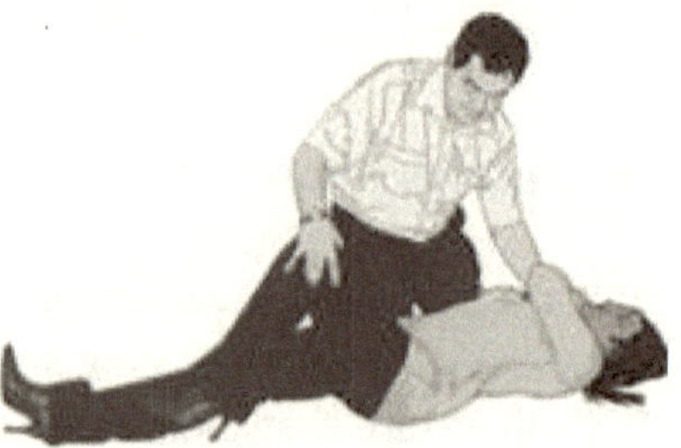

Keeping the back of the casualty's hand pressed against their cheek, pull on the bent knee to roll the casualty towards you on to their side. You can then adjust the top leg so that it is bent at a right angle.

- **Step 4: Ensuring an open airway**

Place the patient's hand under their chin to stop their head from tilting and to keep their airway open. Continue monitoring the patient and if he stops breathing and goes back into cardiac arrest he should be rolled back into the supine position and CPR restarted.

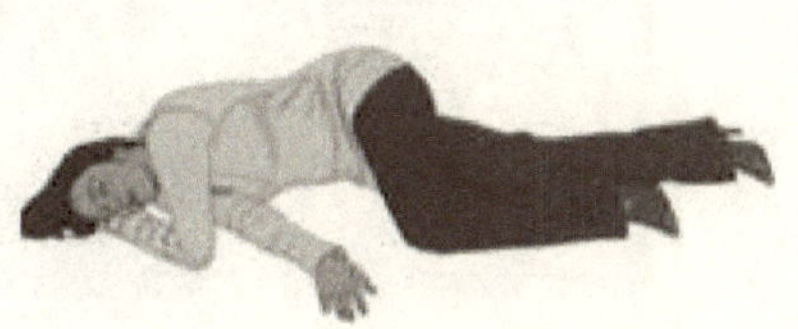

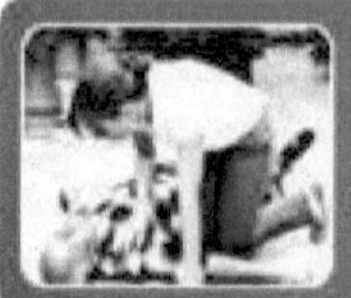

Is the victim unresponsive, not answering to calls, having absent or abnormal breathing?

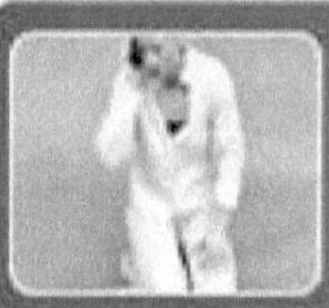

Call 112 Emergency Medical Services

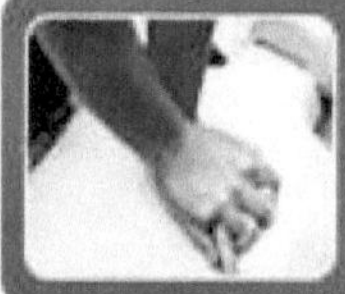

Give 30 high quality chest compressions

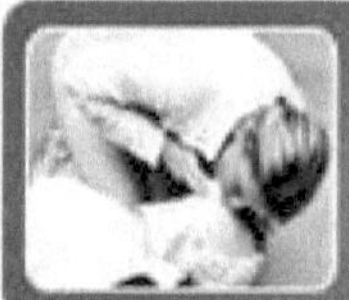

Give 2 effective rescue breaths

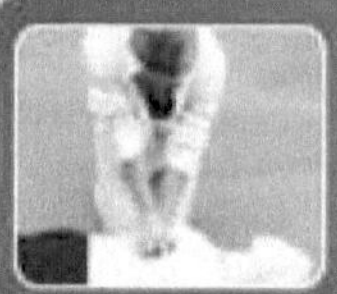

Continue cardiopulmonary resucitation

30 chest compressions : 2 rescue breaths.

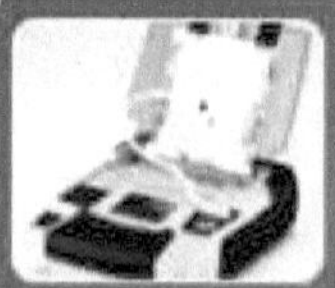

Switch on the AED as soon as it arrives and follow all intructions prompted.

Managing the airway and treating choking [Heimlich manoeuvre]

Introduction

A continuous supply of oxygen is essential for every cell to be able to function properly and remain viable. Once the body is deprived of oxygen for any length of time, then the process of cellular anoxia is established leading to death of cells and failure of organ systems. The regular supply of oxygen to the tissues can be interrupted if the air passages become obstructed. This obstruction can be partial or complete and can affect the upper and/or lower respiratory tract.

Patients requiring resuscitation often have an obstructed airway caused by or the result of unconsciousness. In such circumstances, for the patient to survive, airway management must be rapid and effective. Several conditions can result in airway obstruction of the upper respiratory tract [see Table below]. A stepwise approach to airway management, starting with the simplest and most rapidly applied, will ensure that the airway is secured as quickly and as effectively as possible.

Upper respiratory tract obstruction	Lower respiratory tract obstruction
• The relaxed tongue or epiglottis falling back in the throat in the unconscious patient.	• Excessive secretions in the tracheobronchial channels.
• The presence of foreign fluids, such as blood, vomit, saliva, etc.	• Aspiration of regurgitated gastric contents
• The presence of food.	• Pulmonary haemorrhage
• Foreign bodies, such as displaced dentures, toys, etc.	

Potential causes for Airway obstruction

The commonest situation faced by the First Aider is airway obstruction of the upper respiratory tract linked to the oro-pharyngeal region. In these situations the First Aider is well placed to effectively assist the victim with good manual airway techniques, suction and patient positioning. The well-trained First Aider can also effectively assist cases of laryngeal respiratory tract obstruction using the Heimlich manoeuvre. With the limited means at his/her disposal, the First Aider can do very little to effectively assist in lower respiratory tract obstruction.

Identifying the condition

The first essential step in management is to identify that the victim is suffering from airway obstruction. The principles steps for identifying the condition include:

- **LOOK** – start your assessment by looking for the chest and abdominal movements associated with breathing.
- **LISTEN** – listen for the airflow through the nose and mouth.
- **FEEL** – feel for the airflow through the nose and mouth.
- **TIME** – check the respiratory rate which for an adult at rest should be 12-20 breaths per minute.

Airway obstruction can be complete or partial. In complete airway obstruction, the victim appears to be making paradoxical respiratory effort chest and abdominal movements. Thus, as the patient tries to inhale, the chest is drawn in and the abdomen expands, with the opposite happening during expiration. In partial airway obstruction, air entry is reduced and usually noisy. In upper respiratory tract obstruction, there will be an inspiratory stridor suggesting laryngeal spasm or physical obstruction. Other potential sounds include gurgling – suggesting the presence of liquids or semi-solid material in the airways, such as blood or vomit; and snoring – arising from the airway being partially occluded by the tongue or palate. An expiratory wheeze suggests obstruction of the lower respiratory tract tending to collapse and obstruct during expiration.

Management

Once any degree of obstruction is recognised, immediate measures should be taken to maintain a clear airway. The management plan will depend on whether the obstruction occurs in a conscious or an unconscious patient. A stepwise approach to management will ensure the most suitable method of airway control is achieved.

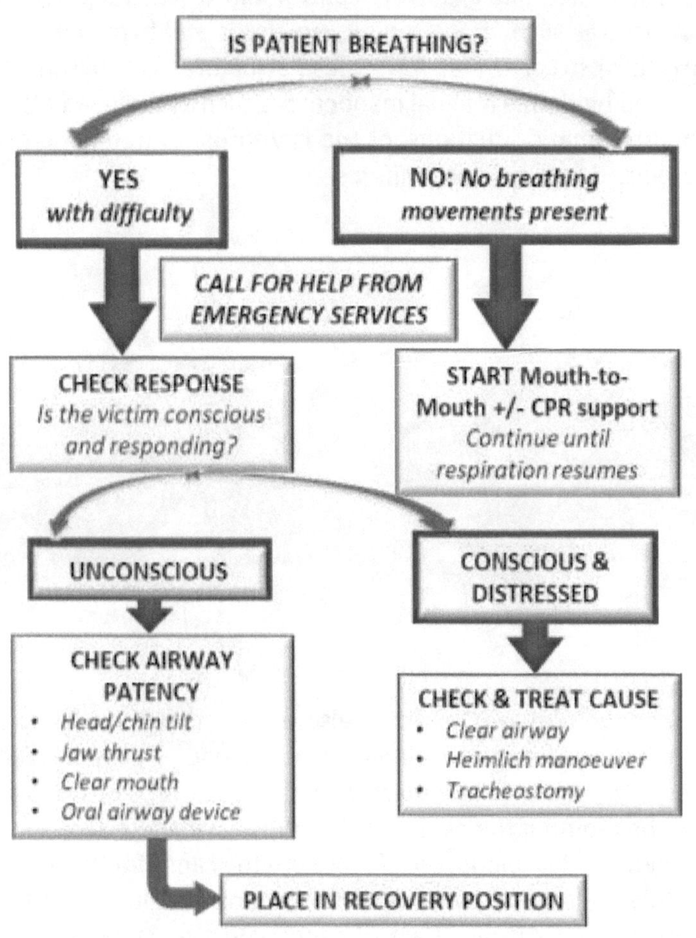

The first step in managing the airway is to ensure that there is no obstruction to the flow of air. Primary attempts at establishing and maintaining a clear airway can include a combination of manual methods and use of airway adjuncts (if these are available). Once the airway patency and spontaneous breathing is restored, the patient should be placed in the recovery position and reviewed regularly.

Manual methods of airway control aim at ensuring that the soft tissue structures such as the tongue, epiglottis and hypopharynx do not fall back to obstruct the airway. These structures can be anatomically repositioned by simple manual manoeuvres such as the head tilt and chin lift in non-traumatic situations, or the jaw thrust in traumatic situations with suspected cervical spine injuries.

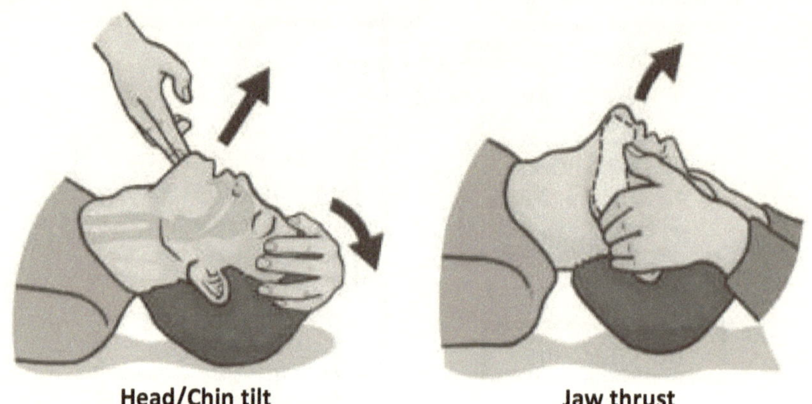

Head/Chin tilt   **Jaw thrust**

Clear the airway: One must also ensure that there is no foreign body/fluids obstructing the airway. Foreign bodies may include food, dentures, toys, etc. Check for these digitally and extract. Do not place your finger in the mouth if the person is rigid or is having a seizure. Fluids may include vomit, saliva, blood, etc. If these are the cause for the obstruction, then simply turn the victim's head to the side to allow drainage while maintaining the jaw thrust. Care of course must be taken in turning the head in cases of suspected head injuries. A Mucus extractor to clear the airway from any fluids within the airway is a useful implement.

Oral airway devices will relieve soft tissue obstruction of the posterior airway by displacement of the tongue and soft tissue anteriorly. They should only be used in the unconscious patient as vomiting, aspiration and laryngospasm may otherwise occur. The airway device may be inserted sideways or upside-down and, once it is well into the mouth, rotated and advanced in to the full position.

Heimlich manoeuvre is a simple technique useful in cases where the individual is choking. If the victim appears to be choking, but can breathe and cough, their own coughing is probably more effective in clearing the obstruction that the aid you can provide.

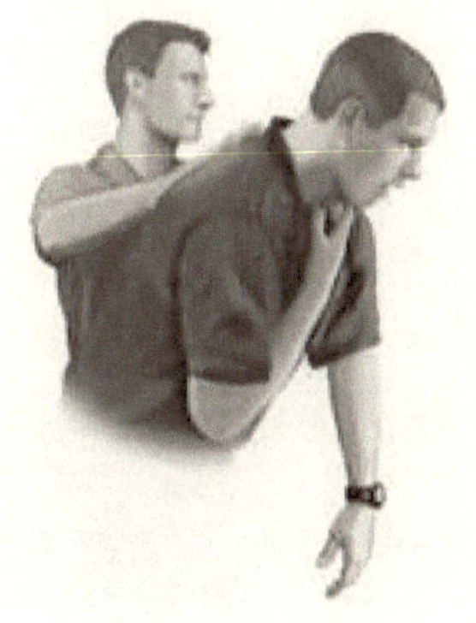

A series of thumps on the back between the shoulder blades may sometimes help dislodge the foreign body enabling the victim to cough it out. Start by leaning the victim forward and delivering four sharp blows to the back between the shoulder blades.

If this does not work, then proceed to apply the Heimlich manoeuvre.

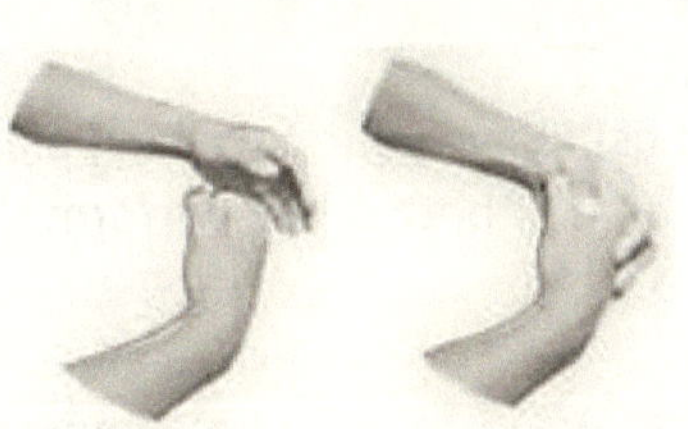

Stand behind the victim. With the victim leaning forward, wrap your arms around the abdomen. Make a fist with one of your hands placing this thumb side in the centre of the victim's abdomen (between the waist and bottom of the ribs). Grasp that fist with the other hand.

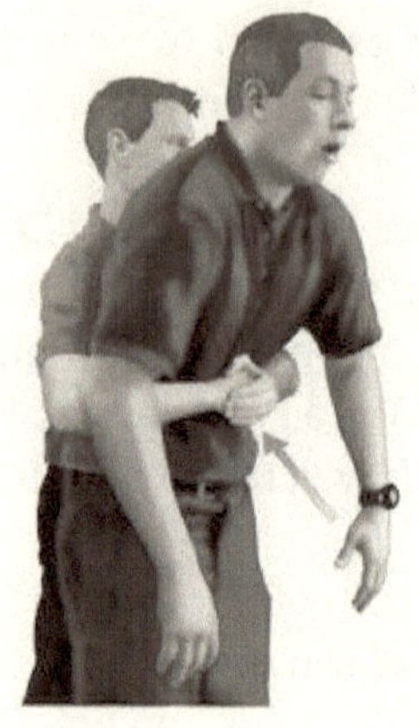

Give five upward thrusts using quick hard movements inward and upwards.

If this does not work the first time, **DO NOT GIVE UP**. Repeat the process starting with the delivery of sharp blows to the back to dislodge the object and then reapplying the Heimlich manoeuvre. Continue repeating the attempts until the victim starts breathing or coughs loudly.

If the victim is obese or pregnant, use chest thrusts instead of abdominal thrusts, placing your fist against the lower part of the chest, where the lower ribs join to the breastbone.

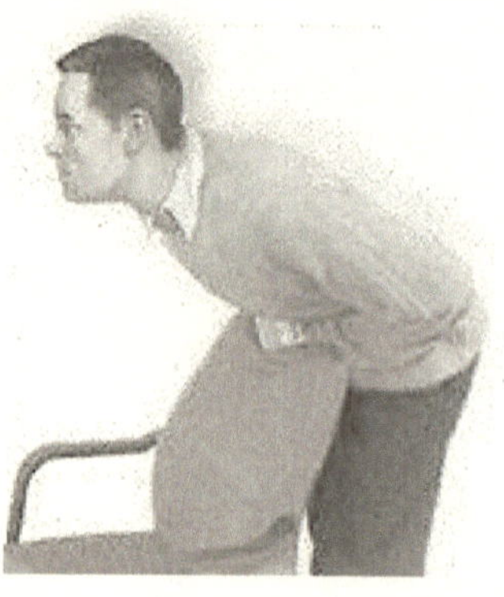

You may be in a position where you are the victim of choking and nobody is available to give you assistance. In these circumstances, you can attempt applying the Heimlich manoeuvre on yourself. Lean forward over the back of a chair and position your abdomen against the top of the chair's backrest. Thrust hard against the back of the chair to compress your abdomen, repeating the thrusts 6-10 times quickly. If no chair is available, an alternative method is to place a clenched fist above your navel and place your other hand over the fist. Using the force of both arms, perform the abdominal thrust on yourself.

Tracheostomy: On the rare occasion when repeated attempts at performing the Heimlich manoeuvre fail, an alternative procedure to bypass the obstruction is the performance of a tracheostomy. This must be considered only in a life-or-death situation where the victim is certain to die without it. Basic instruments needed to carry out the procedure include: a sharp narrow blade (e.g. penknife) and a hollow tube (e.g. ballpoint pen case). These ideally should be sterilized in boiling water, but often there is little or no time to do this.

- Lay the victim on the back with elevated shoulders and the head and neck presenting in a straight line.
- Run the finger down the bonelike projection on the front of the neck (Adam's apple) and identify the smaller projection below this (Cricoid).
- Make a small but deep (about 1-2 cm) incision in the midpoint between the two projections. Twist the blade sideways to open up the cut.

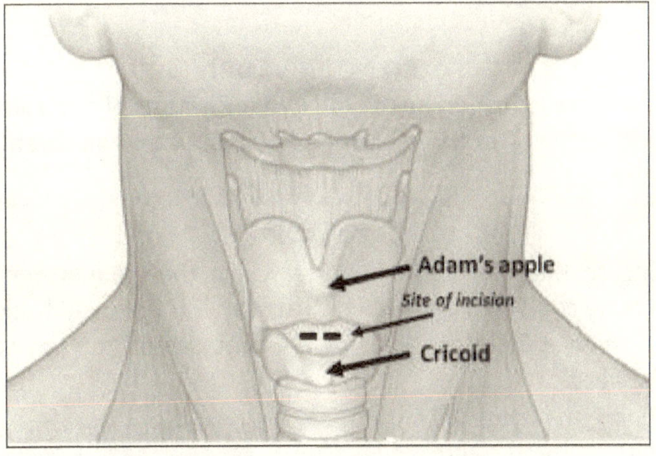

- Then insert the tube into the incision pushing it down to keep the cut open. The tube will allow air to enter the lungs.
- Once in place, secure firmly with adhesive tape or bandage keeping it upright and holding it in place.

Artificial ventilation: Once the airway is clear, if the victim is still not breathing, artificial ventilation must be started. The simplest effective technique to institute mouth-to-mouth respiration. A CPR pocket mask to assist with mouth-to-mouth resuscitation is a useful item if available. A better technique is using the bag-valve mask respirator that consists of a self-inflating bag, oxygen reservoir and non-rebreathing exhalation valve.

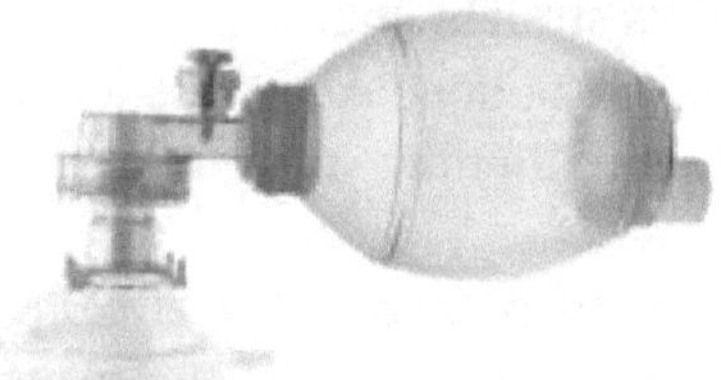

Ambu bag mask respirator

DO NOT GIVE UP!
Artificial resuscitation has saved lives of victims of drowning and hypothermia after three hours without spontaneous breathing.

- Ensure that the airway is clear using the manual methods of airway control or using an oral airway. Tilt the head back slightly to open the airway. Put upward pressure on the jaw to pull it forward.
- Pinch the nostrils closed with thumb and index finger. Place your mouth tightly over the person's mouth. Use a mouthpiece if one is available. Blow two quick breaths and watch for the person's chest to rise.

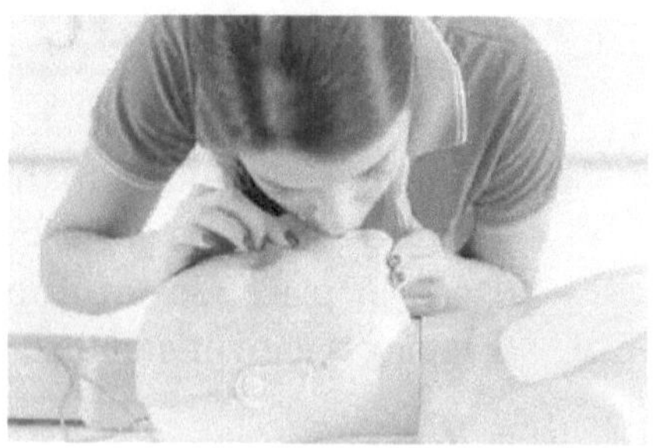

- Release the nostrils. Look for the victim's chest to fall as he/she exhales.
- If using a bag-valve mask, choose the proper size mask for an optimal fit that will provide a good seal around the mouth and nose. The mask is best held in place provider using the "C" shape area between 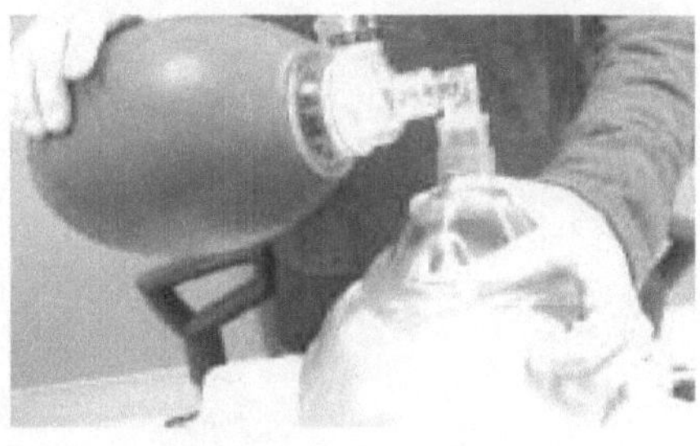 the thumb and index finger, while grasping the mandible with the remaining three fingers, pulling the face into the mask.
- Listen for the sounds of spontaneous breathing and feel for the person's breath on your cheek. If the person does not start breathing spontaneously, keep repeating the procedure.

Controlling bleeding and treating shock

Introduction

The number one cause of preventable death after injury is bleeding. This is due to what is termed as "hypovolaemic" shock. Blood is essential to carry oxygen to all the organs in the body to keep them functioning. Controlling bleeding can save lives and this chapter will demonstrate ways one can control bleeding whether with hands or with a first aid kit if available.

In an average 70 kg person the circulating blood volume is around 5 litres (70 ml per Kg). As the amount of blood is related to weight, the younger and smaller the victim, the more likely for them to lose a serious amount of blood. The more blood lost, the less amount of oxygen that reaches vital organs and the sicker the victim gets. The Table below shows the effects of loss of blood volume in injury victims.

SHOCK	STAGE 1	STAGE 2	STAGE 3	STAGE 4
Blood loss %	< 15%	15% -30%	30-40%	40% +
Blood loss volume (ml)	<750 ml	750 – 1500 ml	1500-2000 ml	>2000 ml
Pulse Rate (beats/min)	<100	100 -120	120 -140	>140
Respiratory Rate (breaths/min)	14-20	20-30	30-35	>35
Blood pressure (mmHg)	Normal	decreased	Very low	Barely or not recordable
Mental state	Normal	Mildly anxious	Confusion/ lethargy	Confused/ unconscious

Shock- signs and parameters

One must, however, keep in mind that the parameters might not give an accurate reflection of the degree of shock in people who are on heart or blood pressure medications or who have heart disease or hypertension. Timely identification and intervention are essential to reduce complications and preserve life.

Bleeding in an injury can be obvious and visible. However, there are situations where the bleeding is internal with no evidence of an external wound. In the latter, large amounts of blood can be lost into the abdominal cavity or chest cavity without signs of external bleeding but still presenting obvious signs of shock. In situations where internal bleeding is suspected, tight clothing especially trousers are best kept on since these may help in diverting blood flow towards the vital central organs.

Vascular injuries can be caused by almost any of the above types of wounds and, depending on the size and nature of the injured vessel, can result in severe bleeding that can be life-threatening if appropriate measures are not taken. Haemorrhages divide into arterial haemorrhages and venous haemorrhages, and the distinction is relatively simple – venous bleeding flow constantly while arterial bleeding spurts out in concordance to the cardiac rhythm.

- In all vascular injuries, the first measure is to stop the bleeding. This assistance must be done as soon as possible with the available means. When the bleeding source is identified, apply direct pressure on the wound to control bleeding.
- When dealing with any body fluids, it is important to keep in mind the risk of transmitting blood-borne infections, e.g. hepatitis or HIV, to oneself. Precautions must be taken to avoid direct contact with blood by the use of gloves [while not ideal, a plastic bag over the hand will also suffice].

Principles of Management of injury causing bleeding

The size of the wound does not reflect the degree of bleeding as a small wound can still damage a major blood vessel with significant blood loss. The Basic First Aid principles should always be followed whenever one is called to tend a victim of an accident that results in a wound with signs of external bleeding.

> **Ensure your own safety**
>
> **A** - **Alert emergency services & call for help from bystanders**
>
> **B** - **Identify bleeding points**
>
> **C** – **Compress & apply pressure to the wound to stop the bleeding.**

- When assessing a victim who is apparently bleeding, it is important to correctly identify the source of bleeding. Remember that the body has a front and a back and some bleeding sources can be in areas not immediately accessible or visible. However, when moving the victim ensure that all other precautions to maintain the Airway with Spinal protection as outlined in other chapters.

- Clothing needs to be opened or removed to be able to visualise the wound clearly, keeping in mind that the victim needs to be kept warm and privacy maintained. Look for and identify "life-threatening" arterial bleeding indicated by spurting of blood, soaking of clothing, pooling on the ground, loss of tissue, and signs of shock as described earlier on.

- Once the bleeding points are identified, once can set about trying to stem the blood flow. To succeed in this one must apply pressure higher than the pressure driving the blood out. Therefore, bleeding from veins needs much less pressure than bleeding from arteries. Direct compression of the wound can be applied by:

- Covering the wound with a clean cloth and applying pressure by pushing directly on it with both hands. Part of the victim's clothing can be used if nothing else is available on site.
- Packing (stuffing) the wound with gauze or a clean cloth and then applying pressure with both hands. This is especially useful in a gaping wound or where there a large area that needs covered. Although tempting, it is advised not to remove the packing to check if the bleeding has stopped until medical care is available.
- If there is a foreign body stuck in the wound, it is important not to dislodge it as it might have been acting as a plug, slowing the bleeding. Pressure then will have to be applied around the foreign body.

Venous bleeding

- Bleeding from veins and capillaries usually occurs in a slow continuous flow and can be stemmed by simple pressure over the bleeding point, with or without a dressing.
- Ideally place a dressing on the wound and maintain firm constant pressure for 5-10 minutes [longer for individuals on any medications or suffering from any medical conditions that delay clotting].
- Resist the temptation to lift and look.
- If blood seeps through the first dressing, place another on top of the first.
- Initially continuous pressure can be applied manually, but for more prolonged pressure the wound site covered with the dressing can be bandaged using a crepe bandage. The bandage will also keep the dressing in place.

Arterial bleeding

- Arterial bleeding is a more serious form of bleeding occurring in powerful rapid spurts.
- Speed in management is of the essence - An arterial bleeding does not leave much time to fetching or look for dressing material or even resort to a first aid kit!
- Minor arterial bleeding may be controlled using a well applied pressure bandage. Bleeding may be controlled or stopped by applying pressure directly in the wound with the thumb.
- Elevate the bleeding part.
- Arterial bleeding can be temporarily stemmed by compressing the artery at a point where this passes over a bony area. When applying such pressure, keep an eye of the wound – if the blood flow is not immediately reduced when applying pressure, you may have not quite found the appropriate pressure point (see figure) and so move the fingers until the right place is found and the blood flow is reduced.
  - Head wound: Press sterile compresses and apply a pressure dressing.
  - Face wound: Covered with several layers of dressings and apply light pressure.
  - Neck injury: Pressing a sterile dressing onto the wound in the hollow between the larynx and the neck muscle.
  - Upper limb injury: Elevate the arm, apply constant pressure on the appropriate pressure point, then cover the wound and apply a pressure dressing.
  - Lower limb injury: Press strongly on the wound and apply constant pressure on the appropriate pressure point, then cover the wound and apply a pressure dressing.
  - With limb injuries, heavy uncontrollable bleeding can be controlled using a tourniquet.

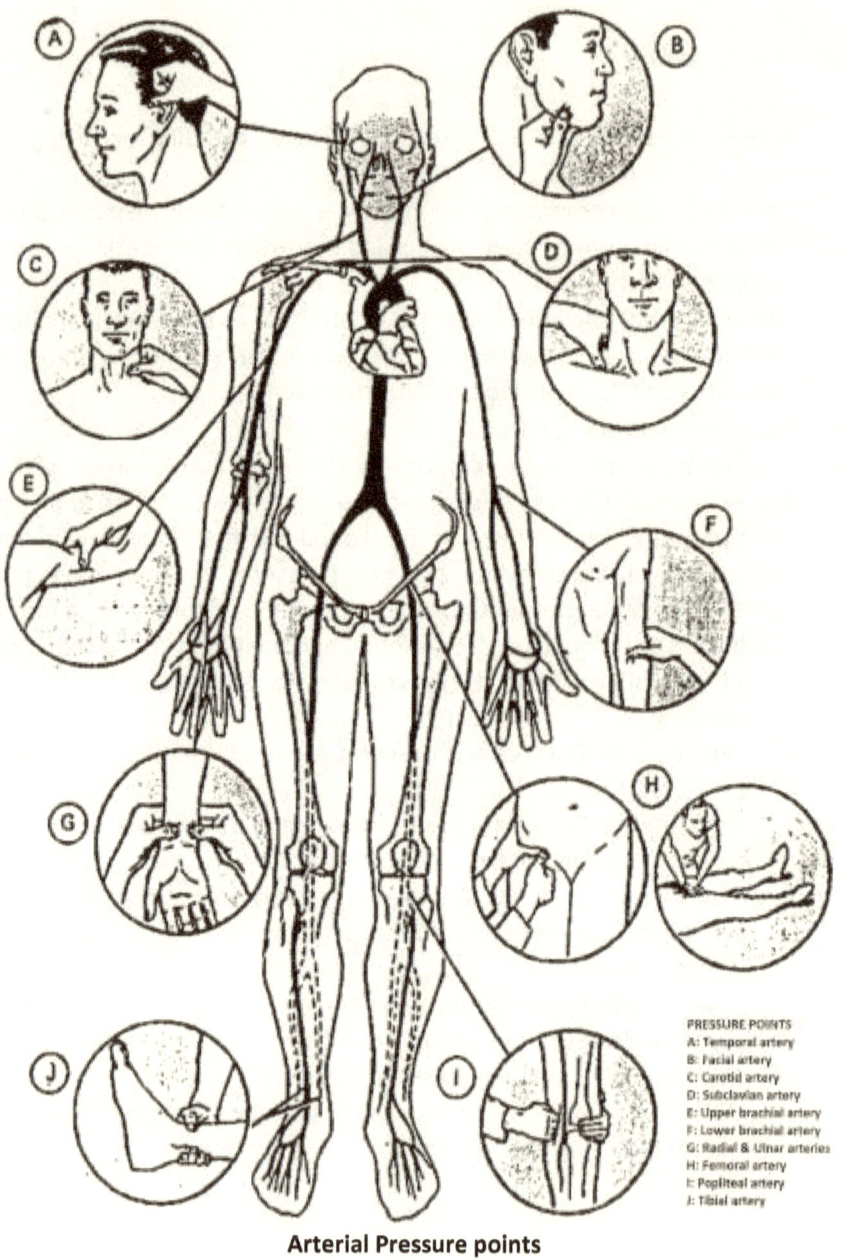

Arterial Pressure points

Use of a Tourniquet

The standard tourniquet looks like a belt that has a ratcheting device or windlass on it that helps tighten the tourniquet as much as needed. It is important to be trained on how to properly use tourniquets as, even when used properly, they can lead to complications. The role of a tourniquet is to completely stop blood from flowing to an area, so it can only be used in limbs when the bleeding cannot be stopped by any other means and the victim is exsanguinating. As it cut off blood flow completely it can lead to complications, therefore it should only be applied for the minimal time possible.

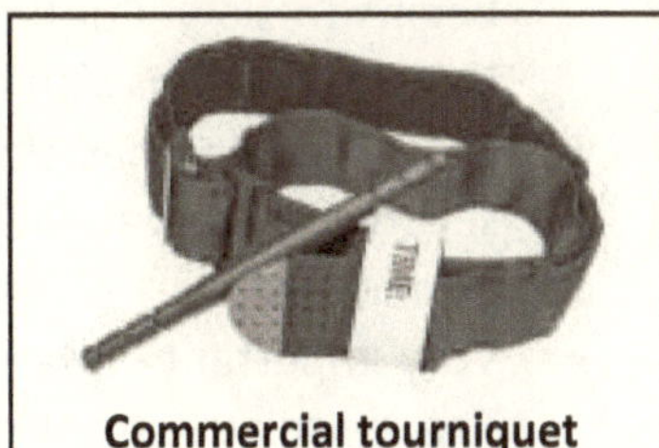

Commercial tourniquet

In cases of severe bleeding, or life-threatening situations, proper use of a tourniquet can stop bleeding and keep an injured person stable until they receive proper medical attention. Tourniquets may be useful in cases such as car accidents, deep lacerations, gunshot wounds, and crushed limbs. If you do not have a commercial tourniquet, you will need to improvise. Tourniquets can save lives if used appropriately.

There are only two places where a tourniquet may be applied: on the upper arm just below the armpit and around the upper thigh. A tourniquet needs to be applied if bleeding fails to slow or stop.

- Forewarn the victim that you will be applying a tourniquet to control the bleeding, as this may be a painful process.
- Cut any clothing near the wound. The tourniquet needs to be applied over exposed skin.
- If a commercial tourniquet is not available, improvise using triangular bandage and a stick to assemble the tourniquet.
- Position the bandage or clothing piece to be used as a tourniquet on the limb about 5 cm [2 inches] above the injury. It is important not to place the tourniquet directly over a joint.
- Make a knot to tie the tourniquet around the limb.

- Next you will need a stick or a similar item to use as a windlass (a lever that is twisted to make the tourniquet tighter).
- Place the windlass on the knot, and then tie the loose ends of the tourniquet around by making another knot.
- Start twisting the windlass to increase pressure. At the same time, you need to observe the bleeding site to note when bleeding begins to slow. Continue twisting the windlass until all bleeding has stopped or is significantly reduced.
- Once bleeding has slowed or stopped, the windlass should be secured to the patient's limb by tying the ends of the cloth to the arm or leg.
- Very important – Mark the time when the tourniquet is applied. The tourniquet must not stay on for more than 2 hours. In the meantime, it should not be loosened or removed, unless the patient is in the Emergency Department.

Pitfalls in tourniquet application:
- Do not hesitate or delay applying a tourniquet – the patient may end up in shock if there is loss of an excessive amount of blood.
- Tourniquet must be securely tightened to actually collapse the arteries. If it is left too loose, then it will serve only as a venous tourniquet leading to continuous bleeding.
- Do not leave the tourniquet on for too long – this can cause permanent damage to muscles, nerves, and blood vessels.
- Use of inappropriate material such as ropes – this may damage skin and cause more pain.

Internal bleeding

Internal bleeding can arise after a violent blow to the body resulting in abdominal or chest organ damage, in association with broken bones, or after deep penetrating wounds. The bleeding is concealed and hence there will be no or little evidence other than systemic symptoms.

The victim will complain of feeling light-headed, restless and faint. On examination, he/she will look pale with cold and clammy skin. The pulse will be very fast and weak.

Effective management is difficult in a Field Emergency situation where one can only apply basic nursing care and hope for an early evacuation. Emergency management would include:
- Lie the patient flat with the legs elevated.
- Keep the victim moderately warm but do not overheat – overheating would result in blood being diverted to the skin reducing further the overall blood volume.

Nosebleed

There are many causes that may trigger nosebleeds. They often are triggered by trauma but may also be a symptom of a medical condition like hypertension. Recurrent nosebleeds without an obvious cause must be reviewed by a doctor since there may be an underlying nasal canal pathology.

Management of Nose Bleeds
- Ask the patient to sit down with the head tilted forward.
- Very important – do not tell them to lean their head back as this can cause blood to trickle down the throat and block the airway. Ingestion of the blood should be avoided, as this can cause nausea and vomiting.
- Ask the patient to breathe through the mouth and pinch the soft part of the nose for 10 minutes.
- Give the patient a clean tissue to catch any blood.
- Cool the neck with an ice pack or wet cloths to attempt constrict the vessels.

- After 10 minutes, release the pressure on the nose. If bleeding restarts, ask the patient to pinch the nose again for another 10 minutes.
- When bleeding stops, ask the patient to keep the head forward while you clean around the nose with warm water.
- Instruct the patient to rest, avoid exertion and avoid blowing the nose to avoid dislodging any clots.
- In case of severe bleeding, or if it lasts for more than 30 minutes, seek medical assistance.

Managing soft tissue injuries and burns

Introduction

Soft tissue injuries can present in various forms and result in a variable number of accident conditions. The commonest forms of soft tissue injury that require first aid attention include lacerations and burns that penetrate the skin's protective cover. Non-penetrating injuries can however also be life-threatening since the trauma caused by the accident may result in cardiac compromise [e.g. electric shock], or promote hypovolaemic cardiovascular shock [e.g. intra-abdominal bleeding after abdominal trauma].

Lacerations

Lacerations and tears are usually the result of sharp object or blunt trauma injuries. Blunt trauma injury causing lacerations may occur following a fall or blunt blow. These blunt injury lacerations typically are found on parts of the body – such as on the head, elbow, knee, palms, and shin – where the underlying bone is only cushioned by a small amount of muscle and fatty tissue. Sharp object trauma lacerations, or stab wounds, are caused by sharp objects penetrating the skin. These may be superficial injuries but, in the case of stab wounds, the injury may be of unknown depth where severity cannot be adequately assessed. Because the depth of such wounds cannot be assessed by simply relating to the visible superficial skin injury, stab wounds can cause life-threatening internal bleeding even in the case of inconspicuous external injuries. In such circumstances, the patient must always be examined in a hospital setting. Penetrating stab injuries include animal bites [dealt with in a separate section].

General measures respecting lacerations

- Control and stop any bleeding if present. This can be generally achieved by elevating the injured limb and applying pressure over the wound preferably using a pressure dressing. If bleeding is profuse, call the medical emergency services for help.
- Maintain a germ-free environment as far as possible. Use the sterile materials from the first aid kit properly unpacking them in such a way that they do remain sterile and ensuring that you do not touch them on the contact surface, but only handle them by touching the edges.
- After placing the sterile dressing on the wound, padding with a second dressing if necessary, secure with an elastic gauze bandage or plaster strips.
- Positioning the victim according to necessity, but the patient should at least sit down – circulation problems often do not occur until a few minutes later.
- Enquire about precipitating events for the injury: Why did the victim injure him/herself? is there a further underlying medical condition that contributed to the injury, perhaps a circulatory problem or hypoglycaemic event contributing to the fall?
- Enquire about vaccination history: Whatever the type of injury, the victim must be asked about his/her vaccination history to ensure adequate cover against tetanus, hepatitis, etc.

Minor superficial wounds – abrasions and superficial lacerations

- After cleaning the skin around the wound with water or disinfectant if available, remove visible dirt and foreign matter such as glass, etc.
- If the wound is bleeding, control the bleeding by the application of a preferably sterile or other improvised available dressing [handkerchief, tissues, etc.] and secure with a bandage.
- The edges of a minor wound can be held together using "butterfly stiches" or cut adhesive plasters.
- Extensive minor wounds may require format stitches to keep edges together, sometimes gluing may be another option. This should be

done within 6 hours in order to promote healing by primary intention reducing scarring.

Large deep wounds

- Gaping wounds are best treated in hospital and usually need formal exploration and management, otherwise there is a risk of poor healing and wide scars – it is best to refer the victim for formal medical care.
- If bleeding from the wound is severe, grasp the sides of the wound. Squeezing firmly together until a suitable dressing becomes available.
- Then apply the dressing and maintain pressure on the bleeding part.
- Cover the dressing with a pad of soft material and secure firmly with a bandage.
- If the bleeding is not completely controlled, apply more dressing or pads.
- If necessary, pressure should be maintained for at least fifteen minutes.
- If anatomically possible, the injured part should be elevated.
- It is generally best to refrain from formally attempting to clean the wound from foreign bodies such as earth, sand, or gravel. This is best done in the hospital. Wiping, brushing, or rinsing may drive the present germs even deeper into the tissue and additionally potentially introduce other germs.
- If the foreign body causing the injury, especially nails, glass or metal splinters, knives, etc., is still stuck in the wound, it must not be removed under any circumstances. Removal risks causing further injury resulting in potential severe bleeding. Simply pad and fix. Do not apply a pressure bandage to such wounds under any circumstances! Simply secure the foreign object with padding.
- If the foreign body is no longer in the wound, it must not be discarded, but must be taken to the hospital for a better assessment of the injury.
- In the case of stab wounds to the abdomen or chest, special care must be taken because of the risk of injury to vital organs such as large

vessels, heart and lungs, liver, and other abdominal organs. In such instances, the victim's vital functions must be closely monitored. In these circumstances, the sooner the victim gets to hospital for formal medical attention, the better.

Burns and Scalds

Burns are often caused by accidents in the home and garden. The most common causes of burn injuries in the home are touching hot stove tops, careless lighting of the barbecue fire with the help of spirit and trying to extinguish burning oil in the pan with water. Children are particularly at risk: on the one hand due to a lack of awareness of danger, on the other hand due to inattention on the part of parent. Hotplate burns are also a significant source of danger for children. Another potential source of burn for babies and young children is being placed very close to an exceedingly hot hot-water bottle without any protective cover. Sunburns are also another form of burn and need to be managed accordingly.

Like burns, scalds are usually caused by accidents in the home and garden: by the carelessly turned-on boiler from which boiling hot water sprays or by the playing toddler who pulls the pot off the stove and douses himself with boiling oil. The difference from a burn is that scalding is caused by contact with hot liquids and burns are caused by "dry" heat.

Major severe burns are life-threatening and must be treated properly. Hospital treatment is necessary in these cases. Burns are divided into three different degrees of severity:
  I.   Mild burns: characterised by a painful red area involving the superficial layers of the skin. This generally heals without scarring, e.g., sunburn.
  II. Moderate burns: characterised by painful redness and blistering of the skin reflecting involvement of deeper layers of the skin. Depending on the severity, scarring may eventually occur.

III.	Severe burns: characterised by destruction of the skin surface with a light-coloured to complete charring appearance (do not confuse charring with traces of smoke). These will cause severe scarring. Skin grafts almost always a necessary part of management.

Burns involving >50% of the body are usually fatal if appropriate medical treatment is not made available in time. The proportion of body area involved can be roughly calculated:

- Head = 9%
- Front of torso = 18%
- Back of torso = 18%
- Genital Area = 1%
- Arms (front & back) = 9%
- Front of legs = 9%
- Back of legs = 9%

The surface area of a child is different proportionally than that of an adult and the above approximations do not apply.

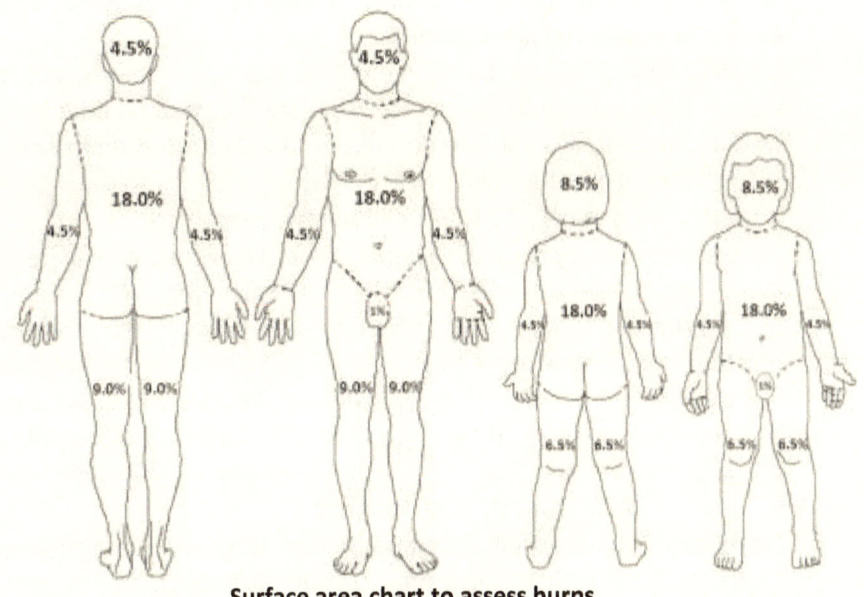

Surface area chart to assess burns

Assessment
When dealing with a burn or scalded victim, assessment of the site of injury is important to assess the potential severity.

R - Recognize the extent of burnt/scalded area
P – Development of pain
R - Reddening of the skin
B – Degree of blistering

Management
- Extinguish any flames using a blanket and remove any smouldering clothes by cutting them off with scissors or knife - undressing takes too long!
- Remove any constricting garments or jewellery – the subsequent tissue swelling will cause these to cause constriction of the affected area.
- Alleviate the pain and cool the heated and injured tissues by immersing in water (at least 15 minutes without interruption). Do not use ice or water that is too cold.
- Do NOT apply 'folklore home remedies', lotion, ointments, etc, to open wound burns – these will contaminate the wound and impede healing. In case of a 1st degree mild burn a dedicated ointment to manage burns may be used.
- If blisters are present, DO NOT deliberately burst them.
- For burns caused by corrosive chemical, wash copiously with water to dilute and wash off the offending chemical. DO NOT attempt neutralizing acid burns with alkali or vice-versa – the chemical reaction will produce more heat.
- Tightly cover the burnt area with sterile dressings, a clean handkerchief, or sheet. If the injured part is the hand or foot, place dressing between the fingers or toes before bandaging the limb – this will prevent them from sticking together.
- Burns cause severe fluid loss and victims are very susceptible to shock. PROVIDE FLUIDS – give small cold drinks frequently, if possible, add half a teaspoon of salt to a pint of water or use a rehydration sachet if available.

- If severely burnt, ensure that the victim is transferred to hospital without delay while controlling for vital functions.

Electric shock accidents

In situations where electrocution is due to a low-voltage (220/230 Volts) domestic current:

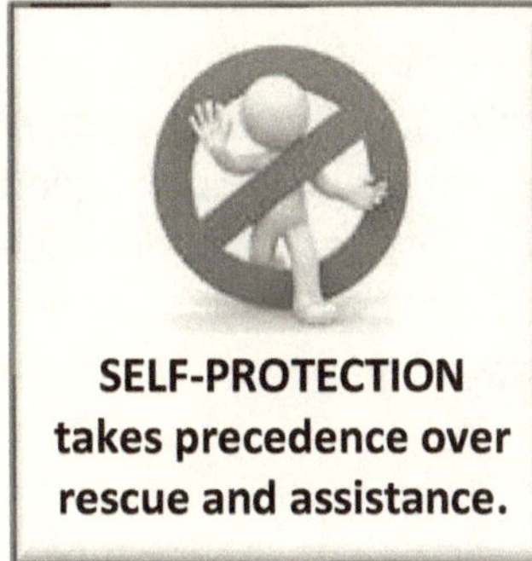

SELF-PROTECTION takes precedence over rescue and assistance.

- Indications that the victim is still in contact with the electrical source include muscle cramps that prevent the victim from letting go of the source → Observe your OWN PROTECTION and do not touch the casualty!
- Switch off the current before attempting to remove the victim from the source. This can be done by pulling out the plug, turning off the main switch or unscrewing the fuse. DO NOT attempt to pull the victim away from the source while current is still on. This will cause you to harm yourself as well.
- If you cannot switch off the current, stand on a dry nonconductive material, e.g., wooden platform, and push or lever the victim from the power source with a dry nonconductive pole or stick, e.g. wooden broom or rolled carpet. Particular care must be taken if poorly insulated cables and/or water are involved, e.g., damaged cable on washing machine, refrigerator, or television coming into contact with leaking water. Never step into the water or wet floor or touch the uninsulated cable.
- Control vital functions and position the victim according to the level of consciousness. If the victim is not breathing and/or has no pulse → start CPR.
- Call for medical assistance. Individuals who have received a supposedly "mild" electric shock must also be reviewed in hospital

to rule out life-threatening cardiac arrhythmias. Life-threatening cardiac arrhythmias may occur up to 24 hours after the event.

- If electric burns are present, manage accordingly – remember that burns caused by electricity are often deep and serious even if not extensive.

In situations where electrocution is due to a high-voltage installations (from >1000 Volts – e.g., overhead lines, industrial machines, transformer stations, overhead lines, electric vehicles and charging stations), the current can only be switched off by specialist personnel such as electricity supplier, fire brigade, or specialised companies. When making an emergency call, it is therefore essential to mention the keyword "high voltage" so that this can be triggered.

- As long as it is not certain that the electricity has been switched off, no first aider should approach the casualty. With high voltage, an "arc", i.e., a flashover, can occur even without direct contact if a certain minimum distance is not maintained. The power supply must be kept at a distance of at least 10 m – 30 m for ends of overhead lines in contact with the ground.
- Be particularly careful in case of high voltage accidents outdoors. Always observe the condition of the ground. Natural soil can conduct the current several metres around the injured person due to normal soil moisture.
- The corresponding confirmation "power switched off" may only be given by the specialists personally present at the accident site. Due to the resulting time delay, these rescue measures may only be carried out by the fire brigade and the rescue service.

Eye injuries

The commonest form of eye injury is the introduction of a foreign body in or blunt trauma to the eye. Penetrating injuries of the eye are more serious with a risk of serious damage or even permanent blindness. Eye injuries, unless minor, should be managed in hospital by an ophthalmologist.

- If the foreign body is small such as a grain of sand, loose eyelash, etc., is situated on the conjunctiva (white of the eye) and does not appear to be embedded, attempts may be made to gently remove the foreign body. Carefully grasp the upper eyelid at the eyelashes and turn it over. If the foreign body is visible, it can be gently removed with the corner of a clean handkerchief moistened with water. If necessary, wash out with water or isotonic saline solution. Do NOT rub the eye in an attempt to displace the offending foreign body.
- If embedded or situated on the iris or pupil, simply apply a gauze dressing or cotton wool pad, secure with adhesive tape, and send the victim to hospital for professional removal. Attempts at removal can result in causing further damage with potential long-term effects.
- If foreign body has a chemical element, whether fluid or solid, then flush the eye with a copious amount of water. Place the victim in the supine position, turn the head to the side of the injured eye and rinse eye only from the inside to the outside with clear water or, if available, eye rinsing solution.
- In situations where there is an increased risk for foreign bodies to be introduced in the eye, it is useful to furnish the site with emergency eye-wash bottles.

- For perpetrating injuries to the eye, do not remove the foreign body. Simply cover with a sterile pad and refer to hospital.

Infected superficial wound

- Wounds can become infected. Local infection can be treated by soaking in hot water in which some salt has been dissolved. Alternative one can apply a poultice to draw out the pus and reduce swelling.
- A poultice can be made from anything that can be made into a paste – potatoes, rice, clay, etc. To prepare the poultice, boil the material you will be using and wrap in a cloth. The wrapped poultice is then applied to the infected area as hot as can be tolerated without it being too hot to cause scalding.
- When pus becomes evident and points, it can be released by opening the wound with a small incision.
- If the infected area appears extensive and especially if it appears to increase through the surrounding tissue, seek medical advice – Antibiotic cover is probably needed.

Managing skeletal injuries including fractures and potential spinal injuries

Introduction

Accident situations can result in excessive strain to the skeletal system causing trauma to the supporting ligament [so-called 'sprains'], to the joint [so-called 'dislocations'], and/or to the skeleton itself [so-called 'fractures']. It may be difficult to identify exactly what one is dealing with → if in any doubt, treat as a fracture.

Fractures: These can be of two types:
- Closed fractures – where the skin overlying the fracture has not been breached; and
- Open or compound fractures – where the sharp edges of the fractured bone has pushed through the skin exposing the fracture to the environment.

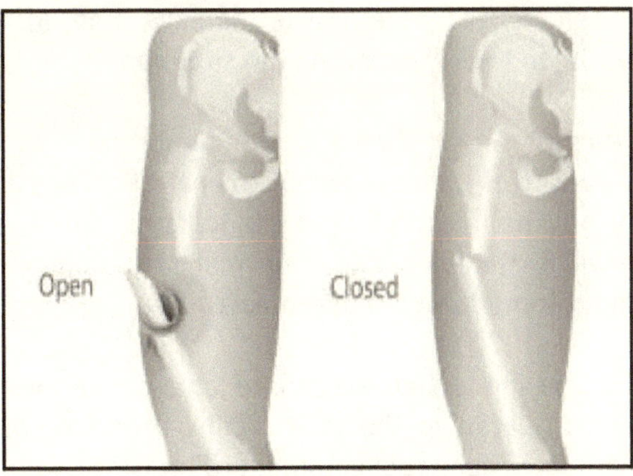

Open and closed fractures

Depending on their severity and location, fractures are generally easily identified. Characteristic features suggesting the presence of a fracture include:

- *PAIN* usually quite severe and made worse on any attempts to move the part.
- *TENDERNESS* on palpation even with only gentle pressure.
- *SWELLING* of the area caused by extravasation of blood into the tissue. Later on, this becomes more evident by the development of bruising. The swelling may complicate the process of clinically identifying the location of the fracture → so it is important to attempt to do this before the swelling develops.
- *DEFORMITY* will result with fractures resulting in loss of skeletal integrity. Always compare the suspect area with the unharmed opposite side. Deformity can exhibit itself as apparent shortening or irregularity of a limb that may be visible or palpable.
- *UNNATURAL MOVEMENT* of a limb in regions far from a natural joint. This may be accompanied by a grating sound. However, **DO NOT** move limbs deliberately to check for any abnormal movement. Beside eliciting severe pain, the forced movement may itself cause more tissue damage and increase blood extravasation thus aggravating the situation.

Dislocations generally occur when a sudden abnormal force is applied to a skeletal joint causing the joint to be pulled apart. Pain and deformity are generally very obvious features with dislocations. Often, the ensuing muscle spasm will fix the joint in an abnormal position making it difficult to reduce without some form of anaesthesia.

Sprains also involve joints and are caused by a sudden wrenching and tearing of tissues related to the joint. Clinical features include pain, swelling, and the subsequent development of bruising.

First Aid management

In an emergency situation where professional help will be on its way, the essential emergency management is to immobilize the affected part as best as possible in the circumstances. First Aid managed should apply the RICE Principle.

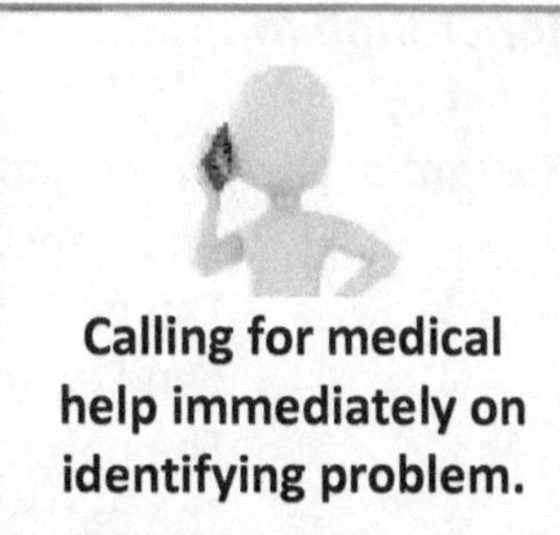

- **R – Rest:** Do not move or try to straited the injured area
- **I – Immobilize:** Stabilize the injured area in the position it was found. Immobilization can be achieved by the use of splints made from any rigid material that may be available. In the absence of suitable material, the injured limb should be strapped to the other uninjured limb or to the body.
- **C – Cool:** Apply a cold pack to the injured area for 20-minute period to help reduce swelling and relieve pain.
- **E – Elevate:** Raise the injured part to help reduce swelling BUT ONLY if the movement does not elicit pain and after the fracture is stabilized.

Principle guidelines for splinting a fracture
- Note whether there is the presence of any open wounds with active bleeding, in which case, these should be given priority.
- In case of a deformity, leave the limb in the same position. Do not attempt to manipulate the fracture. It will cause unnecessary pain and might lead to damage to surrounding tissues, blood vessels or nerves. Corrective attempts should only be carried out after better evaluation in a formal medical setting.
- The injured part may be steadied and supported with cushions or rolled-up clothing.
- If immobilisation by bandages and splints is required, ensure that skin surfaces are separated by soft padding, and that the splints immobilise the joint above and below the site of fracture.

Upper limb injuries

Fracture of the Clavicle (collar bone) – Shoulder or Elbow dislocation
- Call for emergency medical support if:
    - The patient is experiencing numbness or weakness in the hand or arm, and if the hand is cold, pale, or blue.
    - The patient's pulse is weak.
    - The patient is having difficulty breathing or swallowing.
    - The injury was caused by a severe blow.
- Immobilize the upper limb in a triangular bandage (as shown below) until the patient arrives to the Emergency Department.
- Apply an ice pack to control swelling. Do not apply ice directly against skin.
- Do not try to manipulate the arm. This will be managed by medical professionals as required once the patient is at the Emergency Department.

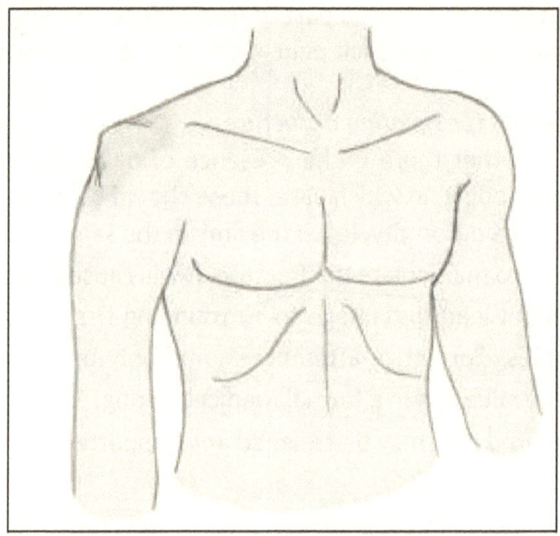

Appearance – dislocated shoulder

Immobilizing dislocations and sprains – tendon rupture
- If in doubt, treat as for fractures. Seek medical attention.
- Rest joint in the most comfortable position.
- Surround it with layers of cotton wool or suitable material and bandage firmly with an elastic bandage.
- With sprains of the upper limb – wrist, elbow, shoulder – support in a sling as for a fracture.

Splinting upper limb fractures
- You will need to improvise a splint depending on your surrounding environment. You need 2 splints, preferably the same length as the injury part of the limb.
- Place the splints on either side of the limb.
- Tie the splint to the injured part of the limb, starting at the bottom and continuing upwards.
- Make sure the ties are not too tight to avoid hindering circulation to the injured limb. You should be able to easily insert 2 fingers side by side between the ties and the limb.

Correctly applying a triangular bandage to make a sling for suspected fractures or dislocations of the upper limb.
- Ask the patient to support the injured arm with the other hand.
- Slide the triangular bandage underneath the patient's arm, with the point of the triangle underneath the patient's elbow of the injured arm.
- Bring the top end of the bandage around the neck.
- Fold the lower end of the bandage up over the forearm to meet the top of the bandage at the shoulder of the injured arm.
- Tie the two ends of the bandage together using a reef knot.
- Adjust the sling to support the arm all the way to the end of the little finger.

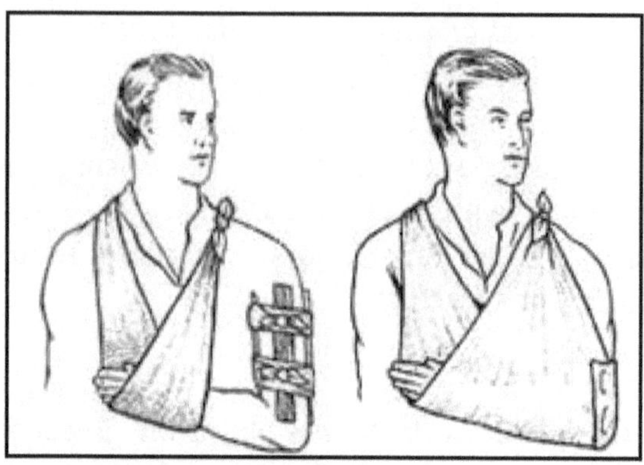

Upper limb immobilization as shown on a vintage triangular bandage

Splinting wrist fractures

- Select a cylindrical object which should be roughly 3 – 4 inches long and 1 – 1.5 inches in diameter (a rolled crepe bandage is suitable for this purpose). This is placed in the hand to add stability.
- Select a straight, rigid, flat object to use as a splint. This could be a ruler, layers of cardboard, sticks, etc.
- Place the splint over the round object in the patient's palm. This needs to touch the fingers on the palmar aspect of the hand.
- Apply a bandage around the splint and the forearm. Then encircle the hand and the splint with the bandage.
- If available, apply ice to reduce swelling.
- Seek medical attention.

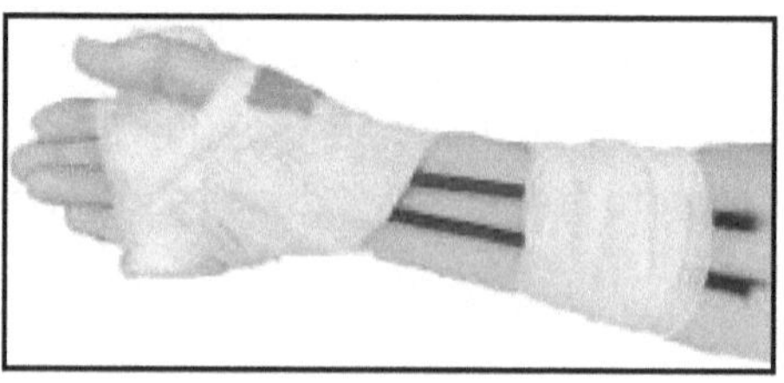

Emergency splinting of wrist fracture

Buddy-taping fingers and toes

Buddy taping is an easy way to treat an injured finger or toe. It involves bandaging an injured finger or toe to an uninjured one. The uninjured finger/toe acts as a splint, and helps to support, protect, and realign the injured finger/toe. It can also help prevent further injury to the digit. This technique should not be used if there are any obvious deformities from the injury, such as a bone at an odd angle. It is important to seek medical advice in case of open wounds that could require stitches, bones visibly out of place, or severe pain.

- Place soft padding between the fingers or toes.
- Wrap the tape around the digits by starting at the base. Wrap the tape 2 or 3 times while using gentle pressure during wrapping without making it too tight.
- After taping, check that the fingers / toes still have good circulation. This is done by pressing the tips of fingers / toes for a few seconds, and then release. If they fill back up with blood within 2 seconds, the wrap isn't too tight. If they remain pale, you need to remove the tape and start over.

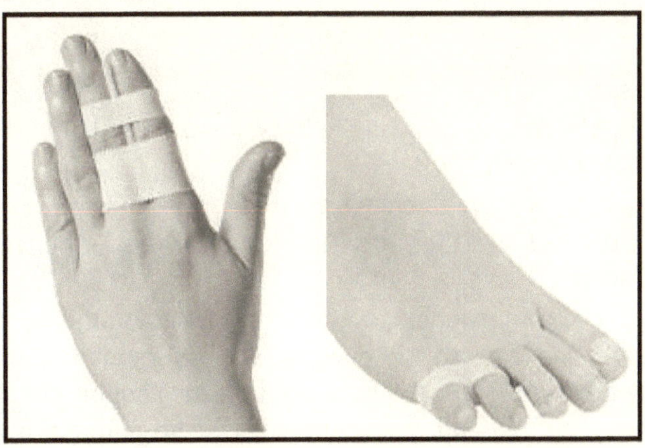

Buddy taping digits

Skier's thumb

Skier's thumb is an acute partial or complete rupture of the ulnar collateral ligament of the thumb following hyperabduction injury.

- Apply ice to the thumb to reduce swelling.
- Immobilize the thumb with an elastic bandage or a brace.
- Seek medical help as soon as possible.

Nursemaid Elbow in children

Nursemaid's Elbow (pulled elbow) occurs in small children after being lifted, yanked or swung by the hand or wrist, or after falling onto an outstretched hand. The radial head (a bone in the forearm) slips out of place. The child may complain of pain at the elbow, cry when the arm is moved or touched, and support their arm with the other arm.

- Do not try to put the bone in place.
- Put the child's arm in a triangular bandage.
- Seek medical attention – the healthcare provider may need to manipulate the arm.

Lower limb injuries

Hip fractures

- Keep the patient lying on the back. Keep the patient warm with a blanket or coat.
- Call for help from the medical emergency services.
- Tie the legs together at the ankles and knees – the legs may be straight or bent.
- Apply a splint extending to the whole length of the injured limb – secure the leg with stiff padding, such as wadded-up blankets or towels, held in place with heavy objects. Padding should extend above the hip and below the knee. If no material is available, place one hand behind the knee and the other hand along the top of the thigh, so your hand is just below the pelvic region.
- If the patient has to travel some distance, immobilise the fractured bone by tying with a figure of eight bandage his feet and

ankles together, then tie together his knees, legs and then the thighs. Finally secure with a fifth bandage the limbs immediately below the site of the fracture.

- Stay with the patient until medical help arrives.

Splinting lower limb fractures
- Note whether the victim is conscious or whether there is the presence of any bone deformations or open wounds with active bleeding, in which case, these issues should be given priority.
- In case of a deformity, leave the limb in the same position. Do not attempt to manipulate the fracture. It will cause unnecessary pain and might lead to damage to surrounding tissues, blood vessels or nerves.
- You will need to improvise a splint depending on your surrounding environment. If you're in the countryside, grab some thick sticks, a hiking pole or a walking stick. If you're at home, you can also use equipment such as a broom. You need 2 splints, preferably the same length as the limb. For even more support, the outer splint can be extended up to the armpit.
- The splints need to be tied together, ideally using bandages. You can also use items such as belts, shirts, or ties to achieve the same results.
- Place all the equipment in place before tightening everything.
- Start by laying the tying item (bandage, etc) under the limb. Place one by the ankle, one below the fracture and one above the fracture. Do not place anything on the knee or around the wound.
- Place the splints on either side of the limb on top of the tying devices.
- Tie the splint to the leg, starting at the bottom and continuing upwards. The ankle strap can also be tied around the foot. This provides additional support, immobilizes the foot, and prevents the patient from moving the ankle, causing more pain.
- Padding can also be placed between the splint and the patient's body for more comfort.

- Make sure the ties are not too tight to avoid hindering circulation to the injured limb. You should be able to easily insert 2 fingers side by side between the ties and the limb.

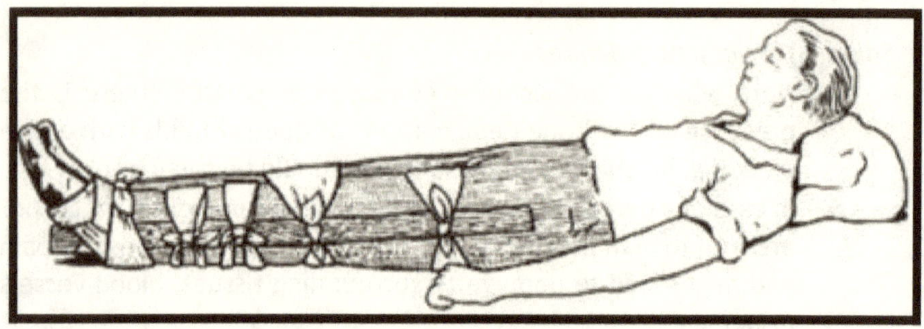

Lower limb immobilization as shown on a vintage triangular bandage

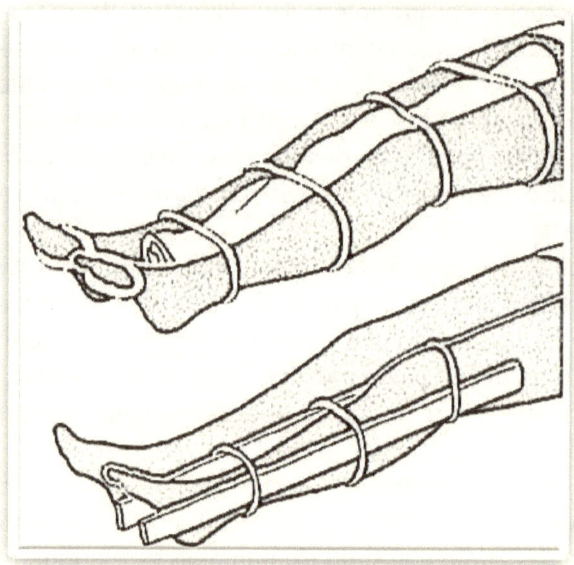

Alternative methods of splinting the lower limb

Immobilizing dislocations and sprains – tendon rupture
- If in doubt, treat as for fractures. Seek medical attention.
- Rest joint in the most comfortable position.
- Surround it with layers of cotton wool or suitable material and bandage firmly with an elastic bandage.
- With ankle sprains, elevate the leg and apply cold compresses.
- Immobilise the foot either by retaining the shoe if this is suitable, or alternatively immobilize with a folded blanket supporting the ankle and foot. DO NOT allow the victim to put weight on the foot.

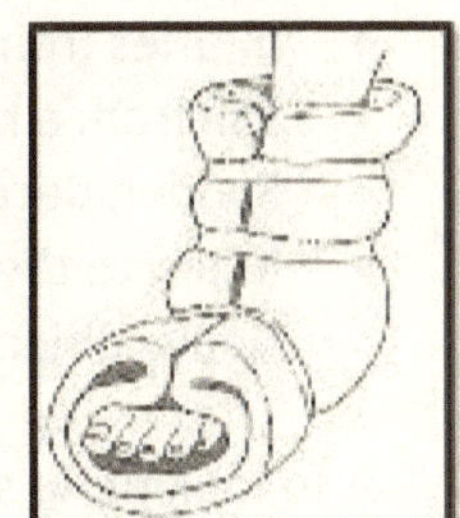

Neck and Spinal injuries

Neck and spinal injuries are particularly dangerous injuries to manage in an emergency situation since any undue movement may result in injury to the spinal cord causing long term serious paralysis. The possibility of a spinal injury must be considered anytime the accident involves the head, face, neck, or back. A potential spinal injury must be suspected whenever the victim complains of pain in the back or neck, with the possible loss of sensation in the lower limbs. Sensation can be tested for by gently touching the limbs – DO NOT use a painful stimulus to check for sensation since this may elicit a withdrawal response by the victim that may jerk the back and cause further injury. You can check for ability to move by asking the victim to wriggle the finger and toes.

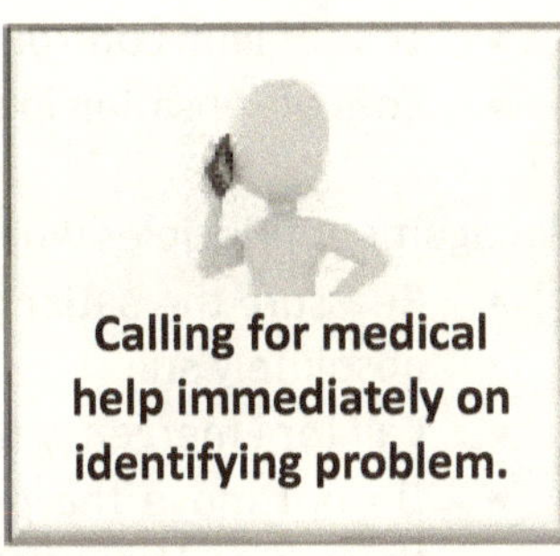

Incidents which could indicate a possible spinal injury:
- Fall from height
- Fall during gymnastics
- Diving into shallow water
- Injuries from aggressive sports activities, such as rugby
- Fall from a horse or a motorbike
- Sudden deceleration in a car
- Injury to the head or face
- Heavy object falling onto the back

What to look for in suspected spinal injury:
- Neck or back pain following injury
- Bruising on the neck or back
- Irregular twist to the spine
- Difficulty breathing
- Loss of bladder or bowel control
- Loss of limb control
- Loss of sensation in the limbs

Management principles when a spinal injury is suspected should include:
- Reassure the patient and advise the victim not to move and to lie absolutely still.
- Call for Emergency Medical assistance.
- Do not move the person from the position he/she is in unless there is an immediate threat to his or her life, such as a fire or if cardiorespiratory resuscitation is necessary.
- If it is essential to move the victim because there is immediate danger, then keep the victim's head and neck supported and in a straight line with the spine while being moved to a safe place. Use the log roll technique ensuring maintenance of spine alignment with adequate personnel to help to turn the victim.
- Try to immobilize the victim and stabilize the neck as much as is possible in the circumstances. In the unavailability of a cervical

collar, place a bag of earth or something similar on each side of the neck to prevent movement.

  o   Kneel by the patient's head – put your knees on the ground for steadiness.

  o   Hold either side of the patient's head and do not cover the ears (rest your elbows on the ground for increased steadiness).

  o   Ensure that you are supporting the head in a way that the head, neck, and spine are aligned.

  o   While you're supporting the patient's head, ask someone else to put rolled towels or clothing on either side of the patient's head.

  o   Make sure you continue to support the patient's head until help arrives.

• If the injury was a result of a diving accident, float the person face up in the water ensuring that the spine is well supported during the process. Do not remove the person from the water – simply wait for help to arrive.

• Continue speaking to the patient – if he/she becomes unresponsive at any point, prepare to follow First Aid principles as required.

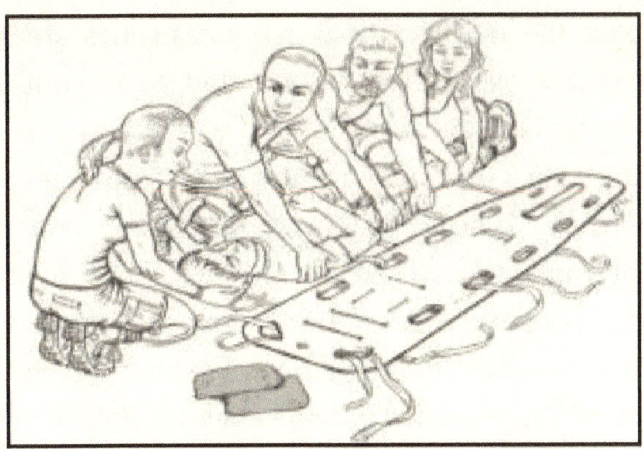

Turning a suspected spinal injury victim

Motorcycle Accidents – Your Role as the First Responder

Riding a motorcycle carries its risks, and it's important to know how to manage the victim of a motorcycle crash if you are the first responder on the scene. High velocity motorcycle accidents can lead to detrimental effects such as head injury, spinal injury, fractures or dislocations, severe wounds, and loss of consciousness.

- Evaluate and secure the scene while walking towards the patient. Never run without being aware of your environment, especially in an area with heavy traffic. This is to ensure that you remain safe throughout the whole time.
- If someone else is accompanying you, it would be a good idea to instruct them to stop oncoming traffic, which might lead to another accident.
- Look for signs of leaking fluid, fumes, broken glass. This reduces the risk of exposing the patient and yourself to further harm in case the vehicle catches fire.
- Get help as soon as possible – call for an ambulance. You will be asked about the location, how many casualties are involved, an estimate of the age of the patient, and also about any obvious injuries that you are observing.
- Most motorcyclists end up hitting their head, especially if it is a head-on collision. When you get to the patient, it is very important to keep him/her still and immobilised. The only exception when you should move the patient is in the presence of danger, such as fire.
- Helmets are excellent stabilisation tools in case of a broken neck. Do not attempt to remove the patient's helmet. Taking off the helmet requires trained personnel (at least 2 people) to keep the neck immobilised, so do not attempt to remove it as it might lead to more harm.

- Speak to the patient to check for responsiveness. Explain the situation and reassure that help is on the way. Most importantly, keep the patient calm by explaining what is going on and reassuring that everything is going to be fine. Ask the driver whether there was a pillion riding with him/her in case there is another casualty who still needs to be located.
- Control any active bleeding by applying direct pressure on the area with pads. Do not remove pressure in case bleeding restarts.
- Remain with the patient until the ambulance personnel arrive on scene.

Amputations

Traumatic amputation is defined as an injury to an extremity that results in immediate separation of the limb as a result of accident or injury. These injuries are classified according to the severity of tissue damage. In complete traumatic amputations, where the limb becomes completely detached from the body, the arteries go into spasm limiting blood loss. In partial traumatic amputations where

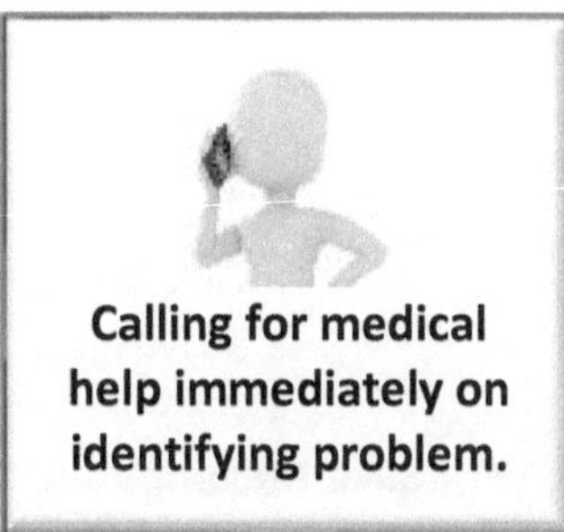

only up to half the injured extremity is damaged significantly is usually associated with more extensive bleeding because not all the blood vessels will become vasoconstrictive. The primary aim of the first-aider is to control bleeding and ensure early transfer to hospital.

Following traumatic amputations, the optimal outcome is that of surgical intervention aiming to reimplant the amputated part. However here the window of opportunity narrow and the decision to reimplant is often influenced by the victim's age and overall health status, the level of the injury, and the condition of the amputated part. It is therefore essential that the amputated part is collected and sent to hospital with the victim in the best condition possible in the circumstances. First aid management points include:

- Control and stop the bleeding
    - Get the injured person to lie down and if possible elevate the injured area.
    - Apply direct pressure on the wound using a sterile dressing. If there is an object in the wound, apply pressure around it, not directly over it.
    - If blood soaks through the dressing, apply another layer over the first one to keep steady pressure. Do not remove the first layer.
    - Use an arterial tourniquet or a compression bandage in case of severe bleeding which does not stop with direct pressure.

- Manage for shock
    - Cover the patient with a coat or a blanket.
    - Talk to the injured to keep him/her calm until help arrives.

- Save the amputated part – in some cases, this can be reattached.
    - If possible, rinse the amputated part with clean water to remove any debris and dirt. Do not use soap or scrub.
    - Place the amputated part in a moist paper towel, and place in a clean plastic bag with ice if available.
    - Send it with the victim to the hospital.

Management of poisoning

Introduction

Intoxication is caused by exposure to a harmful substance by ingesting, injection, inhalation, or any other means. Acute poisoning could involve a wide range of circumstances including:

- Accidental or intentional medicinal drug intake or overdosage.
- Ingestion of household [e.g., detergents] or work-related products [e.g., chemicals, paint, insecticides. Carbon monoxide poisoning can be placed under this category].
- Ingestion of poisonous plants or berries.
- Venomous animal bites or stings.

Poisons can be broadly classified into:

- Corrosive substances usually involving household or work-related products such as acids, bleach, petrol, ammonia, dishwasher powder, turpentine, etc.
- Non-corrosive substances usually involving medications, drugs, plants, perfume, alcohol, etc.

When faced with a case of poisoning, whatever the circumstance, the First Aider should try to establish the nature of the potential poison. If possible, collect any vomit or relevant containers to enable later possible identification of the poison. This information can be helpful in the eventual management of the case. The effects of any poison will depend on the characteristic properties and the physiological/pharmacological effects that the ingested substance has on the body. Symptomatology may take time to develop and therefore medical help should be sought immediately.

The identity of the poison and the size of the dose imbibed may occasionally be difficult to establish with certainty. Fortunately, identification is not generally important to institute the emergency measures needed, unless there is a specific antidote for the poison that is available to the First Aider. Nevertheless, knowing the poison substance helps in anticipating the potential course of clinical events especially in the long-term. It will be of help to the paramedics if you:

- Pass on the container the substance was in or pass on any information you may have regarding what the casualty has taken.
- Let them know when and how much of the substance was taken if you are able to ascertain this information.
- Keep any sample of vomit from the casualty for hospital analysis.

The symptomatology of poisoning is varied depending on the poison ingested. These can include:

- Effects on the gastro-intestinal system: nausea, vomiting, abdominal cramps, diarrhoea, loss of appetite
- Effects on the cardio-respiratory systems: evidence of cyanosis such as purple lips, thoracic pain, cough, difficulty or irregular breathing, palpitations.
- Effects on the nervous system: confusion, vertigo, double vision, somnolence, headache, irritability, numbness and tingling, seizures, loss of consciousness, weakness, urinary incontinence.
- Local effects: skin rashes or chemical burns

Hospital transfer and admission is advisable for all cases of poisoning, even if there appear to be no adverse effects at the time of the encounter. Even if well, the victims may subsequently deteriorate if the poison has a delayed action effect.

Primary Management of poisoning

In cases of poisoning, the First Aider should generally aim at making the victim comfortable and responding to and managing the clinical state that the poison brings about. The immediate intervention to be taken is simply limited to washing away any remaining poison from the lips, face or skin. The victim should not be given anything to drink or eat; vomiting in an attempt to empty the stomach should NOT be induced without medical supervision. Only if fully conscious and co-operative, try to get the victim to rinse the mouth.

First Response basic principles apply with the ABCs of first aid being checked when approaching the victim.

- AIRWAY: Any obstruction in the airway requires immediate attention and needs to be cleared so that asphyxiation is prevented. This is particularly important in the unconscious victim. The victim should be placed on the side and cleared from any foreign body, e.g., vomit, that may be in the respiratory tract. If necessary, the victim can be struck between the shoulder blades to unclog the bronchi. To prevent the tongue from falling back and obstructing the larynx, a chin lift or jaw thrust should be applied and maintained. If available, it may be useful to apply an oropharyngeal airway to prevent obstruction.

- BREATHING: The respiratory function needs to be maintained. Most poisons that impair consciousness are also likely to depress respiration. Many forms of artificial ventilation have been designed, but the most practical in an emergency situation is Mouth-to-Mouth assisted ventilation. Once initiated, artificial respiration should not be discontinued until the victim begins to breath alone or until the medical support pronounces the victim as dead. Should breathing resume spontaneously, the victim still needs to be watch closely since the breathing can suddenly cease again or becomes irregular.

- CIRCULATION: The effectiveness of the circulation system in cases of poisoning needs to be assessed. One should check the victim's pulse and observe the colour and temperature of the hands and fingers. Evidence of cyanosis suggests a poor circulation effectiveness leading to anoxia. Hypotension is a common feature of severe poisoning with substances that effect the central nervous system. A low blood pressure can lead to irreversible brain or renal damage. Hypotension can be managed by elevating the legs of the victim. Other poisons may also directly affect the conducting system of the heart resulting in an irregular heartbeat [arrythmias]. CPR should be initiated and maintained should signs of circulatory insufficiency or failure present themselves.

Other aspects of the victim's physiological functions may also be affected by the poison. These need to be looked out for and managed.

- TEMPERATURE CONTROL mechanisms can be adversely affected indirectly by poisons. Unconsciousness brought about by the poison can promote the development of hypothermia. Its development is not easily identified unless one records and monitors the core body temperature of the victim. It is best that in the presence of unconsciousness, the victim is routinely kept warm with blankets or preferably with a 'space blanket' to conserve heat. However, do not use hot water or heating pad and do not apply anything hot or warm to the limbs. Fever or hyperthermia can also develop, generally in individual who have taken stimulants. In the presence of fever, assessed clinically or with a thermometer, it is important to remove all unnecessary clothing, and sponging with tepid [not iced] water to promote evaporation.

- CONVULSIONS or seizures can be induced directly by the poison or indirectly though the physiological effects of the substance ingested [e.g., hypoxia, hypotension, hypothermia]. Single short-lived convulsions do not require any treatment. However, care must be taken to prevent any potential complications resulting during the convulsion. The convulsing victim should be placed and maintained on the side to ensure that there is less likelihood of vomitus aspiration.

Active general measures to manage poisoning

Active measures to remove the ingested poison can be taken. However, these should be considered only under medically supervised situations and when the poison has been identified. It is usually not practical to apply these procedures in an emergency situation. Measures to remove and eliminate poisons can involve:

- Removal of the poison from the stomach should only be considered if a life-threatening amount of the poison has been ingested within the previous hour. It is essential that the airway is protected and maintained throughout the procedure. Gastric lavage is definitely contra-indicated if the poison is a corrosive substance or a petroleum distillate. Mechanical or pharmacological induction of vomiting is not recommended since it increases the risk of gastric content aspiration and there is no evidence that the procedure reduced absorption of the poison.

- Interfering with absorption of the poison can be achieved by administering oral activated charcoal. This can bind the poison reducing its absorption within the gastro-intestinal system. The sooner it is administered, the more likely is the procedure to be effective. Activated charcoal is relatively safe and is particularly useful in the management of poisons that are toxic in small amounts. It should not be used in drowsy or comatose victims, and when the poison involves petroleum-based products or corrosive substances. An effective 'universal' antidote to help absorb a poisonous fluid can be made up from tea and oral activated charcoal with an equal volume of milk of magnesia if available.

- Methods aimed at active elimination of the toxin are only practical in a hospital environment. These methods furthermore only apply to a limited range of poisons.

- In situations where the poisoning is a result of harmful fumes released in the immediate environment, remove the source of the fumes [gas outlet, car engine, solvent container, etc.], open all windows and doors to ensure an adequate circulation of fresh air. If the victim has no pulse and/or has stopped breathing → start cardiopulmonary resuscitation immediately.

MANAGEMENT OF POISONING

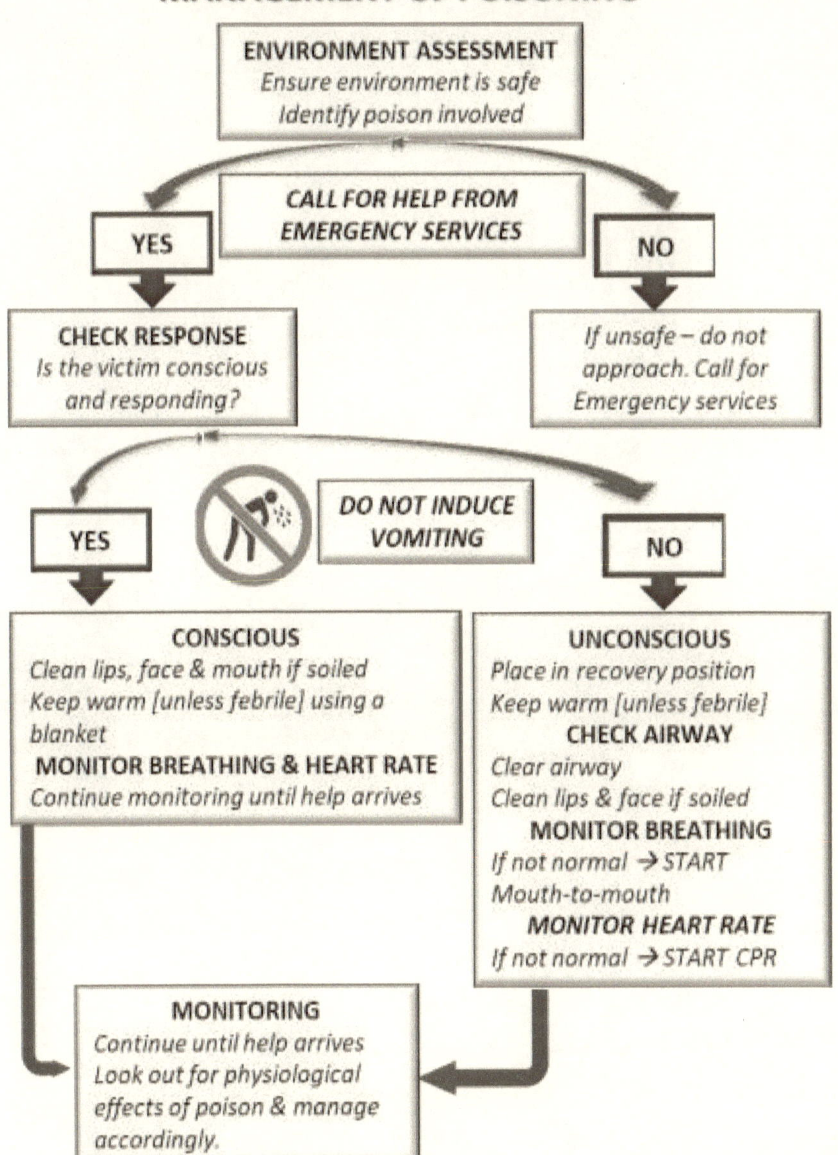

Animal bites or stings

Introduction

Encounters with animals can result in unanticipated injuries brought about by bites or stings. These injuries can be further aggravated by the effects of poisoning or anaphylaxis. The First Aider needs to provide attention to the bite or sting so that the harmful effects of this are minimized and be prepared to deal with the development of anaphylaxis or the effects of poisoning.

Management of human and animal bites

Teeth bites should be considered as deep puncture wounds that not only cause local damage but can also introduce infection, generally causing a local bacterial infection but could potentially transmit other specific infections such as hepatitis or HIV-AIDS in human bites and tetanus or rabies in animal bites. Human bites are generally much more dangerous than dog bites vis-a-vie local infection because of the unusual virulence of the organisms concerned.

The treatment of mammalian bites requires the usual treatment given for puncture wounds with careful cleansing with antiseptics and debridement. Management principles include:

- Wash the bite wound thoroughly with soap and warm water in order to minimize infection. Use a disinfectant if available.
- Raise and support the wound and pat dry with a clean gauze swab or any other suitable cloth. Cover the wound with a sterile dressing or a clean cloth.
- If the wound is deep and bleeding, control the bleeding with direct pressure over the covering pad and raise the injured part. Bandage firmly the injured site. If stitches are needed, these should be kept to a minimum.

- Arrange to send for medical advice if the bite breaks the skin – many will require antibiotic cover. Anti-tetanus toxoid may also need to be given.
- Bites from wild animals and animals not vaccinated against rabies can transmit rabies, the affected person must be treated immediately in the hospital.

The majority of snake bites are not usually serious since most cases are delivered by non-venomous snakes. However, unless the snake is definitely identified as non-venomous, it is safer to assume that there is a risk of snakebite poisoning and manage accordingly. Do not try to kill or capture the snake that bit the victim, but if possible, take a photograph or make a note of the snake's appearance to help with potential identification. Even in areas where venomous snakes are not endemic, it is prudent to manage as a potential poisonous event since the snake may be an escaped exotic species brought to the area as a pet.

Depending on the snake species, the venom may cause local tissue destruction, be neurotoxic blocking nerve impulses thus causing breathing and cardiac problems; or interfere with blood clotting resulting eventually in internal bleeding. The first-aid management of snakebite applies for all species irrespective of the eventual effect of the poison. The main aim of the measures taken should be to prevent the venom from spreading throughout the circulation.

- Reassure the patient and call for medical assistance and urgent transfer to hospital.

- Get the victim to lie down with raised head and shoulders, ensuring that the bitten limb is below the level of the heart.

- Wash away any venom on the surface of the skin, preferably with water and soap.

- Advise the victim not to move the bitten limb to decrease blood flow and venous return to the heart, thus spreading the poison. Consider splinting the limb to immobilize this further.

- Consider placing a restrictive bandage starting some distance above the bite.

- DO NOT apply a tourniquet, slash the wound with a knife or try to suck out the poison. These measures are not of any use in the emergency management.

- If the victim loses consciousness or has trouble breathing, consider starting CPR.

Management of invertebrate animal stings

Invertebrates can also deliver a bite or sting that can result in significant consequences. These bites or stings are usually associated with the injection of some sort of poison that will not only aggravate the pain associated with the sting, but also potentially have serious medical consequences particularly if the individual is allergic to the poison. A large variety of land and marine-living invertebrate species are known to potentially deliver a significant poisonous bite or sting that can cause significant pain and discomfort, and also can result in a serious allergic reaction. Fortunately, few invertebrate species will deliver a poison that is strong enough to significantly affect the victim's health.

It is important that the First Aider becomes familiar with the significant poisonous species in the region. Emergency first aid measures in these circumstances would follow the same principles as those of poisoning. It is important, whenever possible, to identify the culprit species.

Commonly encountered stings are those delivered by bees, wasps, and hornets. For many individuals, a bee or wasp sting is a minor annoyance thought a painful experience. Stings can be fatal in themselves only if occurring in large numbers [hundreds in an adult]. However, a number of individuals may suffer a variable allergic reaction to the inflammatory substance in the sting venom resulting in anaphylactic shock. When stung, the victim will experience pain at the site followed by redness and swelling around the sting.

Preventive measures can be taken to prevent oneself from being stung. Certain types of clothing can serve to protect against stings - white or light-coloured clothing with a smooth finish is less likely to excite bees/wasps to attack; leather is particularly irritating, but the insects will also become disturbed with bright coloured dark rough or woolly material. Bees also seem to become irritated over perspiration odours, perfumes, suntan lotions and hair sprays. It is always best to remain motionless than to try to run away [unless being pursued by a colony of bees or wasps!]. Do not swing at the animal but slowly retreat, with the face protected with the hands. Alternately, just lie face down. There are eight insect repellents for use on skin: DEET, picaridin, IR3535, oil of lemon eucalyptus (OLE), para-menthane-diol (PMD), 2-undecanone, catnip oil, and oil of citronella. By far, the most popular ingredient is DEET. The best prevention however is to avoid disturbing bees or wasps' nests. Wasps are fond of sweet alcoholic drinks, and picnickers should keep their eye out on their drinks, lest they imbibe a wasp together with their cool drink! Being stung in the mouth or throat is associate with local swelling that may be severe enough to cause the airway to block.

The first-aim management of a bee/wasp sting, and also scorpion stings and spider bite, involves attempts to reduce the pain and the development of swelling. Emergency management should include:

- The bee, not the wasp, will often leave its sting sac in the wound; thus, to treat the sting, remove the stinger by scraping it away with a fingernail or the edge of a knife-blade. Grasping it with the fingers or tweezers will only serve to inject further venom into the wound.

- Wash the wound with soap and water and apply antiseptic and a cold compress; ice will help to reduce the swelling. If stung in the mouth, give the victim an ice cube to suck or cold water to sip while seeking medical attention.

- Pain and irritation can be relieved by applying a paste made from either baking soda and water, or meat tenderizer and water. The meat tenderizer - developed to break down protein - also neutralizes the bee/wasp venom. Bee venom is acidic and should be neutralized by the application of ammonia, backing soda or methylene blue. On the other hand, wasp venom is alkaline and requires acid such as vinegar or lemon juice for its neutralization. [Bicarbonate for Bee; Vinegar for Vasp!]. An analgesic-corticosteroid lotion is often useful.

- Monitor the vital signs and watch for signs of an allergic reaction. The symptomatology of anaphylaxis can include generalized soreness and swelling, fever and chills, joint and muscle pain, light-headedness, and bronchial constriction. Other severe reactions include a sudden drop in blood pressure with loss of consciousness, difficult breathing, shock and occasionally death within an hour. Call for medical help immediately if any of these signs start to develop. If available, administer antihistaminic tablets and a pre-loaded syringe of epinephrine to counter the allergic response of the sting.

A number of marine animal species, such as stings from coelenterates (jellyfish, sea anemones, corals) and fish (stingrays, weaver and scorpion fish) are also associated with venomous stings. These injuries generally cause severe burning pain and a red welt - at the site of the sting. With coelenterate stings initial lesions appear as small papular eruptions in one or several discontinuous lines, at times surrounded by an erythematous zone. The papules develop rapidly, and the area becomes red and raised. The papules may vesiculate and proceed to pustulation and desquamation, possibly leaving permanent scars. Some victims suffer from a systemic allergic reaction manifestation including weakness, headache, nausea & vomiting, muscle cramps & pain, lacrimation & nasal discharge, increased perspiration, tachycardia, diarrhoea, convulsions and breathing problems.

Emergency management should include measures to:

- *Remove the remaining tentacles*: Any remaining tentacles stuck to the skin should be removed since these will continue to discharge their stinging nematocysts as long as they remain on the skin. The tentacles should be pulled off or scraped off – not rubbed off since rubbing will cause the nematodes to further discharge their poison. Sea water (not fresh water) should be used to help wash away the tentacles.

- *Denaturing the venom*: Several substances have been advocated as useful to denature the venom in the nematodes – alcohol, ammonia, or vinegar. These should be poured over the site to deactivate the remaining tentacles. The injected venom can be denatured by the application of a warm pack over the sting area.

- *Pain relief*: Various substances have been advocated for pain relief, including baking soda, boric acid, lemon juice, gasoline, alcohol, calamine lotion, and meat tenderizer. A topical corticosteroid can be applied to reduce the inflammatory process.

- *Watch for the development of anaphylaxis*: Monitor the vital signs and watch for signs of an allergic reaction. Institute supportive management for anaphylaxis.

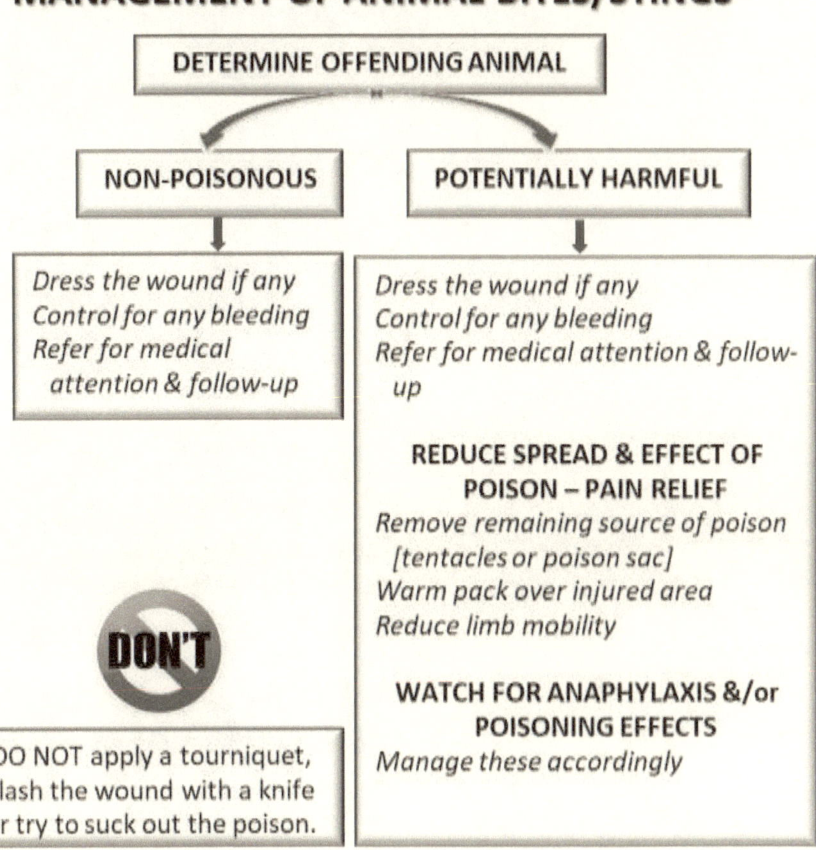

Allergy and Anaphylaxis

Introduction

An allergic reaction is the effect of an immune response activated by a substance such as a particular food (e.g., strawberries), pollen, dust, fur among others. The body would have become hypersensitive to this irritant resulting in an allergic reaction. Common symptoms of an allergic reaction are skin irritation, sneezing, runny or stuffy nose, watery eyes, among other.

Anaphylaxis is a life-threatening reaction to a trigger, most commonly an allergy e.g., eating shellfish or peanuts. It can also occur following the administration of certain medication or following a sting e.g., bee sting. The symptoms of anaphylaxis are more severe and include rash, breathing difficulties, low pulse, shock. Indeed, this is called an anaphylactic shock.

What to do in the presence of anaphylaxis?

1.   Assess the severity of the situation.
   - Is the rash localized?
   - Can the individual speak?
   - Does he/she appear well?
   - Be careful that symptoms of an anaphylactic shock may start as mild and deteriorate rapidly.
   -

2.   Look out for anaphylaxis symptoms:
   - Lightheaded or faint
   - Wheezing
   - Breathing difficulties
   - Clammy skin
   - Fast heartbeat
   - Anxiety and confusion
   - Collapsing or loss of consciousness.

3. If any of these anaphylaxis symptoms are present:
    - Lie the individual down flat, unless unconscious, have breathing difficulties or is pregnant;
    - Call for an ambulance immediately;
    - If the individual is carrying an adrenaline auto-injector (Epi-pen) and you know how to administer it correctly, do so.
    - If you can see the trigger remove it carefully e.g., a stinger stuck to skin.

4. If the symptoms are of an allergic reaction:
    - Make sure that the symptoms do not progressively get severe, in which case follow the anaphylaxis management pathway as indicated in section 3 above.
    - Apply ice to the irritated/ red / swollen skin area. This will help reduce the symptoms and relives the individual.
    - If you have a topical cream containing corticosteroids, apply a small amount on the affected area.
    - Over-the-counter decongestions and antihistamines help to clear the airway and reduce the allergic reaction. Do not take these medications for more than three days.
    - Always seek medical advice if the allergic reaction do not subside or if the allergic reaction was triggered follow the ingestion of medication.
    - Try to identify the triggering allergen to avoid having contact with it again.

Medical Emergencies

Introduction

Medical conditions or their complications can present situations that may require a first-aid response. These conditions may be of no consequence resolving themselves without the need of any intervention; on the other hand, they can result in major health consequences which could have been diminished or prevented with appropriate early action.

Fainting

Fainting is the temporary loss of consciousness that generally lasts a few seconds to a couple of minutes. Before fainting, it is common for the patient to feel lightheaded, weak, dizzy, or nauseous. Some also recall the fading of noises and a sensation of "whiting out" or "blacking out". Most of the time fainting is not of any medical concern; however, it may be a symptom of a more significant underlying problem. Several triggering factors can lead to fainting including emotion, fear, hyperventilation, panic attack, low blood sugar (hypoglycaemia), dehydration, sudden drop in blood pressure, standing up too quickly, physical activity in hot temperature, coughing hard, straining during bowel movement, and after consuming alcohol or drugs.

What to do if someone faints?
The prime goal is to encourage blood flow to their heads. There are two possible ways to achieve this:
1. Lie down the individual on the ground and raise the feet above the level of the heart.
2. Alternatively, have the individual sit down on a chair with the head between the knees.

Other important aspects of first-aid management include:
- Loosen any restricting clothing such as collars, belts, etc...
- Keep the faint individual resting for at least 10 to 15 minutes.
- A cool cloth around their face or neck will help, as will a cool water to drink.

When to call for medical assistance?
In the majority of cases, the individual will very quickly regain consciousness and would require no further assistance. Medical assistance should be called when:

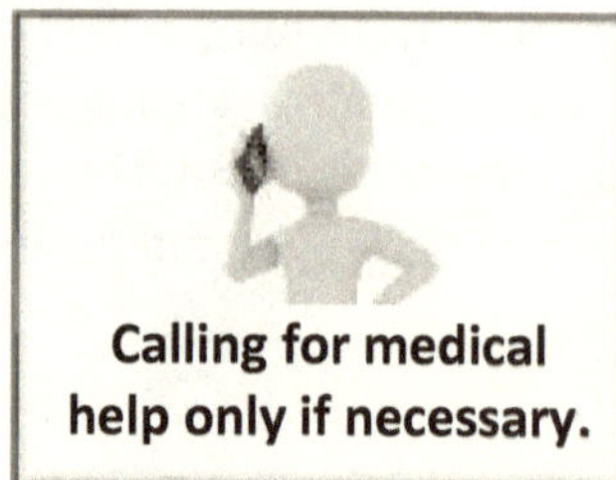

- If the person is not breathing,
- If the person is jerking or shaking – this may be a fit or a seizure,
- If the person cannot wake up after 1 minute,
- If the person, on falling, has got hurt badly.

Seizures

There are several different types of seizures. These occur following a burst of uncontrolled electrical activity between the brain cells that leads to temporary muscle tone or movements abnormalities e.g., twitching, stiffness, limpness. Abnormal behaviours, state of awareness and sensations can also be experienced.

What are the symptoms that suggest a seizure is occurring?
- Falling
- Drooling or frothing at the mouth
- Uncontrolled muscle spasms
- Clenching of teeth, biting of tongue
- Sudden rapid eye movements
- Unusual noises e.g., grunting
- Losing control over bladder or bowel

- Sudden mood changes
- Loss of consciousness and confusion

What should the first aider do in the occurrence of a seizure?
- Do not move the person unless he/she is in danger such as being near a hot cooker or in a busy road.
- If possible, try to place the person on his/her side and place a cushion under the head.
- Loosen any tight clothing around the neck.
- Note down the time of the seizure.
- When the convulsions stop place the person in the recovery position.
- Stay with the person and talk to him/her calmly until recovered – do not allow the person to drive after a seizure.

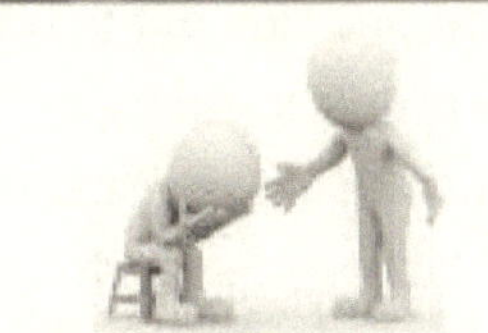

Stay with victim until seizure ends and person is fully awake.

When to call for medical assistance?
- If the seizure lasts for more than 5 minutes,
- If the person does not regain full consciousness,
- If multiple seizures occur without regaining consciousness,
- If the person got hurt during the seizure,
- If you know that this is the first occurrence of a seizure.

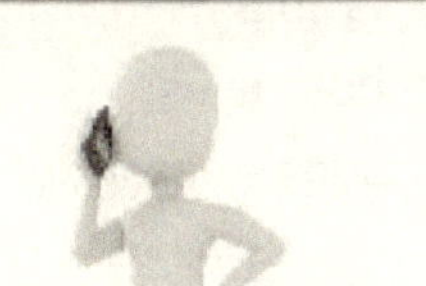

Calling for medical help only if necessary.

Stroke

There are two different kinds of stokes: (i) thrombotic – when a blood vessel in the brain is blocked by a blood clot, and (ii) haemorrhagic – when a blood vessel in the brain ruptures and bleeds. Both types of stroke lead to lack of adequate oxygenation to the brain. This causes the brain cells and tissues get damaged causing these to die within minutes, leaving permanent effects.

What are the symptoms that suggest a stroke is occurring?

- Weakness in the face, arm, leg on one side of the body,
- Trouble speaking or understanding speech,
- Slurring of speech,
- Confusion,
- Trouble walking, loss of coordination or balance,
- Dizziness,
- Problems in vision in one or both eyes,
- Sudden onset of severe headache.

> **FAST acronym**
> F – Face: numb or drooping on one side
> A – Arms: numb of weaker on one side
> S – Speech: slurred or garbled
> T – Time: if YES to above, time to call for help.

How should the first aider respond?

The person requires urgent medical attention. Call immediately for an ambulance. The earlier the person reaches the hospital, the better the chance on timely medical intervention improving the overall long-term prognosis.

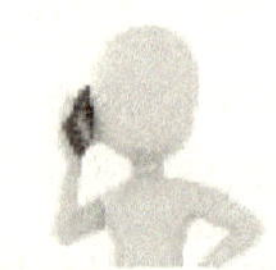

Calling for medical help immediately on identifying problem.

Cramps

A cramp is an involuntary contraction of a muscle on its own. There is usually the formation of a hard lump in the muscle with localised pain i.e., the contracted muscle. Unless the muscle has been strained, a cramp occurs because the muscle has been overused or fatigued, or else because the body is dehydrated. Sometimes it is an indication that the body lacks appropriate amount of electrolytes such as magnesium or potassium. Cramps typically occur in the back of the lower leg (calf area) or the thigh. However, other bodily areas where cramps can occur are arms, hands, feet, and abdominal wall.

What should one do if cramp occurs?
- Stop the activity that induced the cramp.
- Relax the cramping muscle by lightly stretching the muscle and gently holding that stretch.
- Massage the affected muscle.
- After stretching the affected muscle, heat pads can also be applied to the area.
- If the muscle cramp occurred in the middle of the night, one can simply stand up and slowly put on weight on the cramp leg to push the heel down while stretching the muscle out.
- If cramps are continuous and repetitive, it is advisable to seek medical care, as medication in the form of electrolyte supplements may be required.

Headache

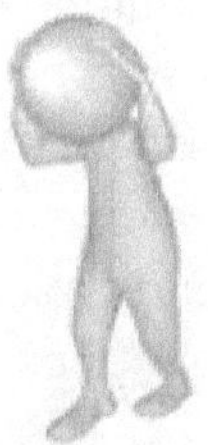

A headache is pain or discomfort that is felt around head and neck. There are various types of headaches and causes. The three most common types of headaches are: Migraines, Tension headaches and Cluster headaches.

A: Migraine

A migraine is a very severe headache with a throbbing or pounding pain, usually affecting one side of the head. This type of headache tends to disturb the daily routine. In severe forms, the individual may complain of nausea and vomiting, with sensitivity to light and sound, in conjunction with the headache. Visual disturbances including zigzag lines, flashing lights, stars and spots can also be present.

What should one do in the presence of a migraine?

The individual should stay in a quiet dark room and take pain killers. Start with 1g paracetamol, however in severe migraines, ibuprofen, or any other kind of NSAID may be need, provided these medications are not contraindicated for other reasons. If the pain does not subside after a couple of hours or symptoms increase, seek medical attention, especially if this is a new migraine occurrence.

B: Tension headache

A Tension headache presents as a dull aching sensation over the head. One may also feel sensitivity or tenderness around the scalp, forehead, neck, or shoulders. This type of headache is usually triggered off by stress.

What should one do in the presence of a tension headache?

The use of over-the-counter pain killers usually relieve this type of headache. If the pain persist it is advisable to seek medical attention.

C: Cluster headache

A cluster headache typically occurs around or behind one eye or on one side of the face, characterised by severe piercing and burning pain. Additional symptoms may include redness, swelling, flushing, and sweating on the side of the cluster headache. Eye tearing and nasal congestion can also occur on the same side of the headache. This type of headache usually occurs in series which can last from 15 minutes to hours and typically occurs at the same time every day. As one headache series disappears, another one will follow.

What should one do in the presence of a cluster headache?
If this is the first episode of encountering such pain, it is recommended to seek medical attention. Those that have been diagnosed with this kind of headache will have a management plan set up by their doctor.

Heat-related illness – Fever – Hypothermia

Heat-related illness can manifest itself as a consequence of a notably hot environment without adequate acclimatization. The manifestations can range from simple prickly heat to heatstroke. Fever can accompany heat-related conditions, but generally presents itself when there is an underlying pathology such as infection.

A: Prickly heat
Prickly heat [or miliaria] can occur when people are exposed to very hot conditions without acclimatization. The heavy sweating, couple usually with friction by clothes, produce blockage of the sweat glands resulting in an uncomfortable skin irritation. Babies and young children are particularly susceptible.

What should one do in the presence of prickly heat?
The best management is to remove the clothing and washing the region with cold water followed by a change of dry clothes. Simply drinking more fluids is likely to aggravate the condition since sweat produced cannot be lost if the gland is blocked.

B: Heat clamps – heat exhaustion
Heat clamps affecting muscles are the first signs of heat exhaustion and results from imbalance of the body's electrolytes following excessing sweating as a result of exposure to high temperatures and humidity. The symptoms include muscle cramps, weakness, dizziness, shallow breathing, and nausea-vomiting. Depending on the severity, the victim can deteriorate to become delirious or unconscious.

What should one do in the presence of heat exhaustion?
The best management is to rest and drink water with rehydrating salt dissolved in it. Propriety sachets of Oral Rehydration Therapy [ORT] are available and it is a useful practice to include these in first aid kits especially in particularly warm countries.

C: Heatstroke
Heatstroke is the most serious consequence of overexposure to the sun's heat. This results in features of a hot dry skin with a flushed face and development of fever. It may be accompanied by a severe headache with vomiting, and possibly the development of loss of consciousness. The skin may show signs of sunburn. The victim may complain or sore eyes.

What should one do in the presence of heatstroke?
In such a scenario, the temperature needs to be brought down slowly.
1. Lay the victim in the shade elevating the head and shoulders.
2. Remove outer clothing.
3. Cool body by wetting underclothing with tepid [not cold] water and fanning.
4. If conscious, give water to drink preferably water with ORT.
5. When temperature returns to normal, replace clothing.
6. In the presence on skin blistering from sunburn – avoid further sun exposure, cover blisters with a dressing and give pain killers if necessary. Do not burst the blisters since this will increase the risk of infection.
7. If eyes are sore – rest in the shade and cover eyes after washing with water. Protect the eyes with dark sunglasses to reduce the glare.

D: Fever
Fever occurs when the body temperature is higher than normal i.e., above 37°C (98.6°F). This is a sign of an underlying problem, usually an infection. Fever is usually associated with several symptoms: chills, sweat, flushing, aches and pains, headache, dehydration, lack of appetite and feeling weak. Fever or pyrexia can be classified as (i) Low-grade or (ii) High-grade fever depending on the temperature reading. A low-grade

fever is usually a body temperature between 37.1°C and 38°C (98.6°F and 100.3°F). High-grade fever is an oral temperature above 38°C (100.3°F). The high-grade fever requires medical attention if the oral temperature is 39.4°C (103°F) or above in adults, for children over 3 months old with a rectal temperature of 38.9°C (102°F) or above while for babies under 3 months old with a rectal temperature of 38°C (100.4°F) or above.

What should one do in the presence of a low-grade fever?

In such a scenario it is not recommended to bring down the temperature too rapidly. The presence of low-grade fever could aid combating the underlying infection. However, taking regular paracetamol (every 4 hours) is recommended. Keeping hydrated and cool, while taking it easy and resting, are also recommended.

What should one do in the presence of a high-grade fever?

In a high-grade fever it is essential to keep hydrated, so one should consume plenty of fluids such as water, juices, or broth. Keeping cool is important, so wear light clothes, sleep with a light blanket, and take a lukewarm bath. Taking it easy and resting is also important. Over-the-counter medications such as paracetamol, ibuprofen can be taken to help with lowering down the temperature and to relieve associated aches and pains. However, in the presence of a high-grade fever it is recommended to seek medical help since antibiotics may need to be prescribed if a bacterial infection is causing the fever.

When to call for medical assistance?

If accompanying the high-grade fever there is the presence of any of the following symptoms, one should go seek urgent medical assistance. This particularly applies for children.

- Rash that does not fade when pressed against a glass
- Bothered by light
- Stiff neck
- Having a fit for the first time
- Pale, blue, or blotchy skin, tongue, or lips
- Unusual cold hands and feet
- Feeling drowsy and hard to stay awake

Additional symptoms in children/babies include:
- Does not stop crying or is extremely agitated
- Not responding normally or show no interest in normal activities or to eat
- Difficulty to breath

E: Hypothermia

Hypothermia occurs whenever the body is unable to generate heat fast enough as it loses it. The body eventually loses the ability to rewarm itself. This results in a temperature drop below normal values. It can be brought about by exposure to wind, rain and low environmental temperatures, but also as a response to medications or poisons. Children are particularly vulnerable to hypothermia. Hypothermic

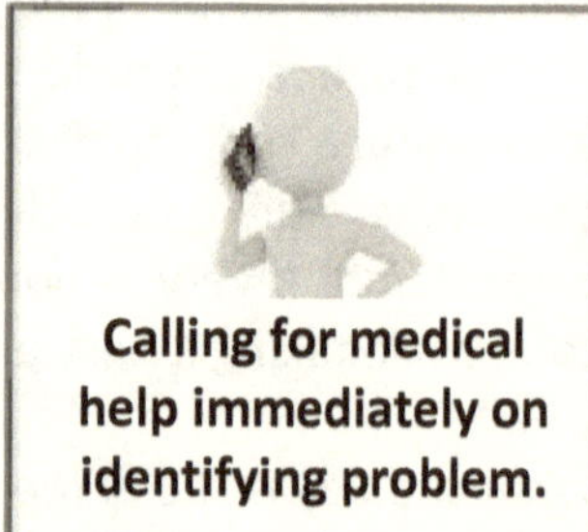

Calling for medical help immediately on identifying problem.

individuals will show increasing lethargy with poor response to questions or instructions, and loss of coordination. They may exhibit uncontrolled fits of shivering.

What should one do in the presence of hypothermia?

1. Prevent further heat loss providing shelter from weather, replacing wet clothing with dry. A foil blanket will help conserve body heat. Insulate from the cold ground by placing a blanket below. Limit movements to only those that are necessary. Don't massage or rub the person. Excessive, vigorous or jarring movements may trigger cardiac arrest.
2. Place in a horizontal position and cover with layers of dry blankets or coats to warm the person. The head should also be covered leaving only the face exposed.
3. Avoid fast external heating since this will drive cold blood into the body core aggravating the condition. Do not apply a warm compress to the arms or legs. Only apply a warm compress to the neck, chest wall or groin. Do not apply direct heat such as hot water, a heating pad or a heating lamp to warm the person. The

extreme heat may damage the skin but can also cause irregular heartbeats.

4. Continuously monitor breathing. If breathing has stopped or appears shallow, begin CPR immediately.

Diabetic emergencies

Diabetic emergencies can present in two major scenarios, either in association with a low blood glucose level (hypoglycaemia) or a high blood glucose level (hyperglycaemia). Both can have serious consequence; however hypoglycaemia presents the major emergency situation since delay in control may have serious life-threatening consequences.

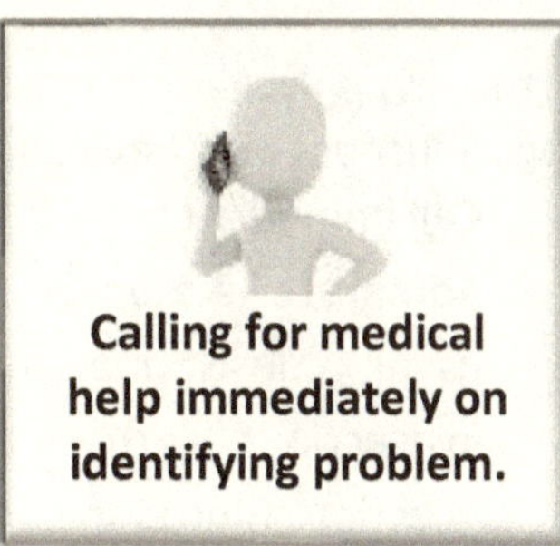

A: Hypoglycaemia (Low blood sugar)
Hypoglycaemia occurs when the blood sugar level decreases below the normal level. This is common occurrence among the diabetes population especially those on medication that increase the insulin levels or those that skip meals or exercise more than usual.

The following are typical symptoms of low blood sugar:

- Sudden mood changes
- Unexplained fatigue
- Sudden nervousness
- Shaking
- Hunger
- Pale skin
- Dizziness
- Blurred vision
- Rapid heartbeat
- Seizure (severe cases)
- Loss of consciousness (severe cases)

What should the first aider do in a hypoglycaemic attack situation?
- Advice the individual to sit down.

- Have them drink or eat 15 grams of easily digestible carbohydrates, which includes:
  - 1 tablespoon of sugar dissolved in water
  - 1 tablespoon honey
  - Half a cup of regular soft drink or juice
  - 3 or 4 glucose tablets or hard sugary candy
  - 4 or 5 salted crackers

If the hypoglycaemic attack is severe where the individual is losing consciousness or is having a fit:
- Call immediately for an ambulance.
- Administer a glucagon injection if available. The glucagon kit will usually consist of a syringe, a vial of powder and a vial of liquid. The instructions in the kit will give details of how to mix these for injection. Glucagon can be injected into the arm, thigh or buttocks. When administering glucagon, put the patient into the recovery position (on their side) to aid their breathing and protect against chocking should the patient vomits.
- DO NOT given anything by mouth in the unconscious individual due to the risk of choking.

B: Hyperglycaemia (High blood sugar)
Hyperglycaemia occurs when the blood sugar level increases above the normal level and stay high for a period. This is the underlying pathology of diabetes. A hyperglycaemic state is usually silent until complications set in. Those suffering from Type 1 diabetes are at risk of developing Diabetic ketoacidosis (DKA) if the blood sugar is too high for a long time. On the other hand, those suffering from Type 2 diabetes may be at risk of Diabetic Hyperglycaemic Hyperosmolar Syndrome (HONK)

Diabetic ketoacidosis (DKA)
This happens when the blood sugar is very high, and ketones start to build up in the body. DKA can develop quickly and is a medical emergency.

The following are symptoms of DKA:
- High blood sugar and urine ketone levels
- Extreme thirst
- Frequent urination
- Vomiting or nausea
- Confusion
- Flushed face
- Fruity-smelling breath
- Abdominal pain
- Fatigue
- Rapid breathing
- Dry skin and mouth

It is important to call for the ambulance immediately. If untreated DKA can lead to a coma and death.

Diabetic Hyperglycaemic Hyperosmolar Syndrome (HONK)
HONK occurs when the blood sugar level is very high, and the body tries to get rid of the excess sugar through the kidneys. However, if the individual does not drink enough fluids to replace the fluids being lost through urine, the blood gets concentrated (hyperosmolar). This causes water to be drawn out of organs including the brain. This is a medical emergency and needs immediate care.

The following are symptoms of HONK:
- Increase urination
- Excess thirst
- Dry mouth
- Nausea
- Confusion
- Cramps
- Speech impairment
- Hallucinations
- Fever
- Vision loss
- Shock (if untreated – severe case)
- Coma (if untreated – severe case)

Mental health crisis

Mental health crisis can arise from various conditions or after certain emotional triggers. A mental health crisis may be arising from depression, anxiety, post-natal (after delivery of a baby) crisis among other situations. This may lead to suicidal idealisation, which must be considered and managed as an emergency needing urgent attention.

It is important to show support and understanding towards the individual experiencing such crisis events, while making sure that they do not harm themselves or others. It may be a good idea to reach out for help such as their doctor or local clinic. Such decisions should be taken with the consent of the affected individual unless they are going to harm themselves or others. Additionally, it is very important not to blame or shame them for their thoughts and actions. Criticizing vulnerable individuals will only serve to worsen the crisis and their reactions.

Hyperventilation – Panic attack

Hyperventilation occurs when breathing occurs at a very fast rate so the oxygen – carbon dioxide balance is disturbed. In hyperventilation, carbon dioxide is breathed out more than oxygen is breathed in, leading to a low carbon dioxide level. This O_2/CO_2 imbalance causes narrowing of the blood vessels and disruption of the blood flow to the brain causing light-headedness and a feeling of tingling in the fingers as well as around the mouth. In severe cases, loss of consciousness can occur. Hyperventilation is usually associated with stress, fear, phobias, and panic attacks. However, it may also be associated with emotional states such as anger, anxiety, and depression.

What to do in a hyperventilation scenario?
The key is to try to keep calm and increase the carbon dioxide level in the blood. The following techniques can be used to treat acute hyperventilation:

- Breathe slowly through a paper bag (important to use a paper bag and NOT a plastic bag!)
- Breathe through pursed lips
- Hold the breath for 10 to 15 seconds at a time
- Breathe into the belly rather than your chest

Identifying the trigger for such an episode is important to avoid having similar episodes in the future. If these episodes are occurring frequently, medical attention should be sought.

Asthma & Croup

Asthma occurs due to a chronic inflammatory process in the passageways of your airway, affecting the ability to breath.

Asthma symptoms vary but the most common include:
- a persisting dry cough,
- wheezing,
- difficulty breathing and chest tightness,
- difficulty to talk,
- fatigue.

What to during an asthma attack?
If this is the first asthma attack, seek medical help immediately.
If the person is a known asthmatic, an action plan should have been developed with the doctor and usually involves the using the rescue inhaler (salmeterol inhaler). If usage of this fast-active inhaler does not provide relied for at least four hours, or fails to improve any symptoms, then need to seek immediate medical help.

Croup is a viral condition that targets children under the age of 5 years, causing swelling around the vocal cords. Affected children present with a bad cough that sounds like a barking seal and breathing difficulties. Other symptoms include fever, hoarse voice, sneezing and running nose. These children require immediate medical attention especially if breathing is being affected.

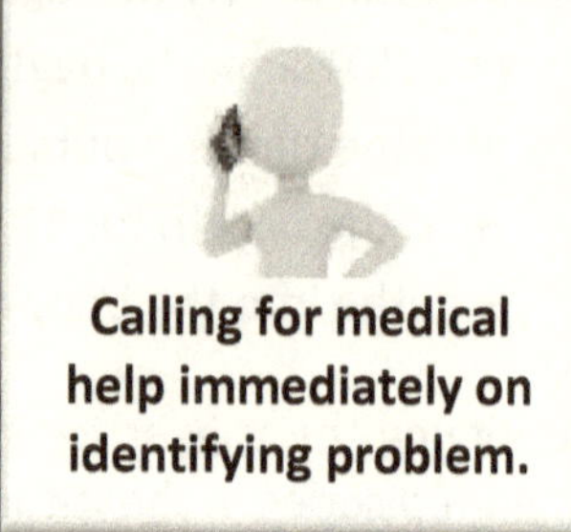

Calling for medical help immediately on identifying problem.

Angina & Heart attack

Angina occurs when there is a reduction in the heart blood flow, resulting in chest pain. This is usually triggered following emotional stress or physical activity including going up the stairs. Such chest pain is an indicative sign that you should speak to your doctor or cardiologist due to a potential underlying heart problem.

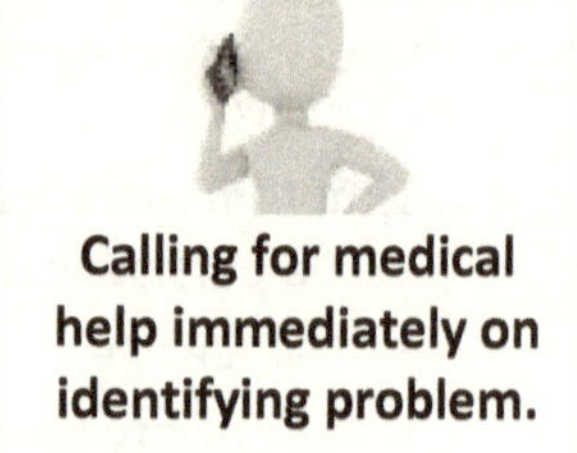

Calling for medical help immediately on identifying problem.

Angina can be divided into two forms:

(i)   stable angina – where the chest pain is induced by a stressor and once the stressor is eliminated, the pain subsides. Indeed, the episode typically lasts around 15 minutes; and

(ii)   unstable angina – this is sudden pain that gets worse over time, which may lead to a heart attack. Both type of anginas may present with several associated symptoms including shortness of breath, fatigue, nausea, dizziness, sweating and anxiety.

What should one do in the presence of an anginal episode?
If this is the first episode, it is important to seek medical attention immediately. If the person has a history of stable angina, his doctor might have prescribed nitro-glycerine spray or sublingual pills to take during such attacks. In such cases, if the pain does not subside after taking this medication or the episode of angina are frequent, then it is important to seek medical attention. If experiencing sporadic angina episodes, it is essential to flag these episodes during the frequent medical follow-ups that one should be attending. In the events of unstable angina i.e., persistent chest pain, it is advisable to seek medical attention immediately.

A heart attack occurs when the blood supply to the heart is cut off leading to parts of the heart's muscle to begin to die. The following are typical "warning" symptoms of a heart attack:

- Central chest pain with or without radiation to the left upper limb (arm) and left jaw
- Sweating
- Shortness of breath
- Nausea
- Fatigue
- Dizziness / light-headedness

In this situation immediate medical is required. Call for urgent medical assistance.

Abdominal pain

The abdomen is the area between the end of the ribcage and the pelvic region. Pain occurring in this area can be achy, dull, crampy, intermittent, or sharp. This could be arising from inflammation or diseases of the underlying organs (small and large bowels, stomach, spleen, kidneys, liver, gallbladder, pancreas, appendix).

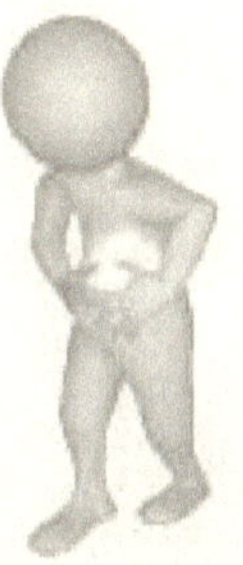

When should one seek immediate medical care?

If the pain is very severe that does not allow one to sit still or else have the urge to curl into a ball to feel comfortable. Additionally, medical attention should be sought in the presence of these associated symptoms:

- High-grade fever (>38.33°C / 101°F)
- Blood in stools
- Persistent vomiting and nausea
- Vomiting of blood
- Yellow eyes or skin
- Severe tenderness or swelling of the abdomen
- Difficulty to breathe

Medical help should also be sought in the event that the abdominal pain is not as severe as discussed above, but it lasts more than 24 hours or if any of the following associated symptoms are present:

- Vomiting
- Prolonged constipation
- Fever
- Loss of appetite
- Dysuria (burning sensation with urine)
- Weight loss which is not explained

Obstetric Emergencies

Introduction

The pregnant woman is subject to a variety of conditions whose consequences can range from causing a minor discomfort to life-threatening situations. Because of the special circumstances of the pregnant state, it is always best to seek medical advice as soon as possible, especially when potentially life-threatening conditions present themselves.

Minor conditions

The pregnant woman is subject to a variety of minor though potentially disturbing symptomatology resulting from the physiological and anatomical changes that take place during pregnancy. It is important that medical advice is sought about the condition if this persists and before resorting to over-the-counter medication.

- *Morning Sickness*: The commonest disturbing symptomatology affecting about half of all pregnant women during the first three months of pregnancy is that of nausea and vomiting, generally worse on an empty stomach. These symptoms generally subside after the third month of pregnancy but may right through pregnancy. Self-care management will include having frequent, small meals instead of a few heavy meals, starting with a dry breakfast. It is important to maintain good hydration, especially in the summer months. Imbibing sparkling water with a slice of lemon may be useful. If the symptoms are very severe and persistent and the woman is not able to keep any fluids or food down, then it is important that medical attention is sought. Anti-emetic medication may be prescribed with good effect, but if the problem persists, hospital admission may become necessary.

- *Heartburn*: Another common gastric problem is that of heartburn, generally presenting itself In later pregnancy since it is contributed to by pressure on the stomach by the enlarged uterus. Self-care management involves having frequent small meals, and not lying completely flat on the bed. The symptoms can be reduced by using antiacids, preferably in suspension.

- *Syncope – fainting*: Temporary loss of consciousness may occur as a result of a drop in blood pressure. The physiological decrease in blood pressure that occurs as a result of the normal physiological processes accompanying pregnancy can be made worse by dehydration and salt loss especially in warm summer months and by prolonged standing in a warm environment. The effects of a low blood pressure with be augmented by a relative hypoglycaemia. Syncope can be prevented by drinking plenty of fluids throughout the day, eating frequent small meals and snacks to avoid hypoglycaemia, and avoiding extremely warm environments and prolonged standing. Management involves allowing the individual to lie down in the left lateral position and elevating the legs. Always ensure that there are no problems with the airway whenever one is dealing with an unconscious individual.

- *Lower limb cramps*: Lower limb cramps can be quite frequent and severe. These are generally associated with dehydration reflecting electrolyte imbalance. Electrolyte-containing rehydration sachets may help prevent cramps from happening. Supplementary calcium tablets may also help. Other preventive measures that can be taken include attention to diet ensuring that sufficient calcium-rich foods, such as milk and milk products, are taken, and not wearing high-heeled shoes. When they occur, management simply involves massaging the affected calf or foot and walk around for some time once the pain has reduced.

Remember that persisting pain in the calf could be a symptomatology of the more serious deep vein thrombosis, and therefore medical attention should be sought if the pain persists or is accompanied by any shortness of breath.

Potentially life-threatening conditions

A number of pregnancy complications can become potentially life-threatening. In these circumstances, there is very little that the First Aider can do with the limited resources available to him/her. In these situations, it is important to immediately call for medical assistance.

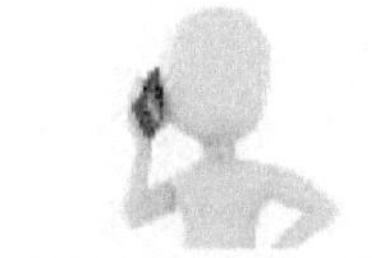

When calling for medical help in cases related to a pregnancy, remember to request a midwife's attendance.

- *Vaginal bleeding*: An episode of vaginal bleeding can occur at any time during the pregnancy. In the first six months of pregnancy, vaginal bleeding can lead to a miscarriage; in later pregnancy may reflect a variable degree of placental separation. The severity of the situation is related to the degree of bleeding that is taking place. One must consider also the emotional stress the mother undergoes at the thought of potentially losing the child. The bleeding may be compounded by severe cramp-like pains in the lower abdomen and the development of haemorrhagic shock. The First Aider must immediately call for medical help, assist the patient to rest in a comfortable position preferably lying down with the legs raised, and continuously reassure the patient that help is on the way. Continue observing the patient while waiting for the ambulance to arrive since her condition may deteriorate. If the patient complains of mouth dryness, one can moisten the lips with water but avoid giving any food or fluids because an anaesthetic is likely to be needed on arrival in hospital.

- *Eclampsia*: Eclampsia is the onset of seizures (convulsions) in the latter part of pregnancy. It is usually associated with the development of hypertension during pregnancy. The condition can herald significant organ failure leading to death of both mother and child. Timely medical support is essential to prevent complications. The First Aider must therefore ensure that medical assistance is immediately called. It is important not to restrain or attempt to hold down the person during the convulsion. In the interim, management should concentrate on reducing the risks inherent in a convulsing patient:
    - Preventing choking: Start by loosening any clothing around the person's neck and place the person in the recovery position (on the side).
    - Protect from self-injury: Move sharp objects, such as glassware or small furniture items, away from the person.
    - Ask bystanders to give the person room.

Childbirth situations

- *Childbirth*: The onset of labour can occur at any time during pregnancy and can initiate in any circumstance. The onset of labour is marked by the development of lower abdominal cramp-like pains occurring at regular intervals and possibly rupture of the amniotic membranes. This will evidently create a sense of excitement mixed with anxiety in the mother and the people around her. There are a number of problems that can occur during childbirth and very little that a first aider can do except stay with the mother and keep her calm until an ambulance arrives. Fortunately, childbirth usually takes several hours, and it is only in exceptional cases that a birth takes place before it is possible for professional help to arrive.

The First Aider must therefore:
- Reassure the mother and others that help is on the way and that you will stay with her.
- Make the woman as comfortable as possible.
- If the woman starts feeling the urge to bear down and push, then is likely that the delivery process has reached the second stage of labour and delivery is imminent. In this situation, one should:
a. get the woman to assume a suitable comfortable birthing position either sitting with knees drawn outwards, or alternatively, in a crouching position helped by a helper.

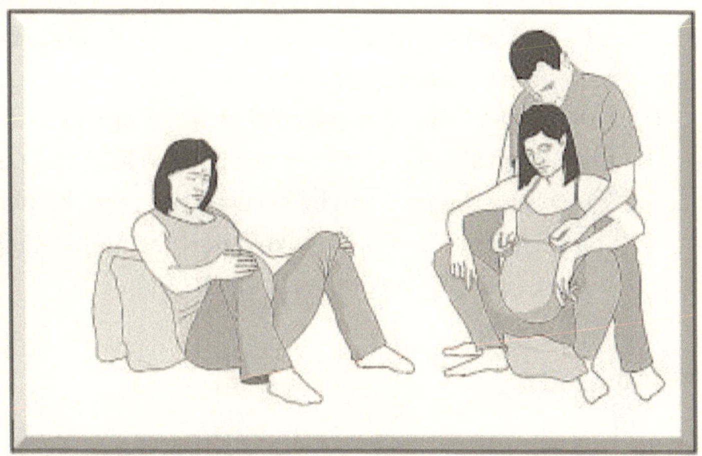

b. advise her not to stop pushing and to pant hard with each contraction to slow the baby's progress down the birth canal, and rest between contractions.
c. remove her clothing sufficiently to expose the birth canal, but ideally cover the thighs and the pelvic region with a blanket – this will help the woman feel less exposed to onlookers.

d. When the head is delivered, tear any membrane covering the baby's face,

e. check whether the umbilical cord is wound round the neck – in which case ease it over the head,

f. then support the baby's head in the palm of your hands, and as the shoulders appear support the body under the armpits and lift towards the mother's abdomen.

g. Once the baby is born, hold it with the head placed lower than the body to clear any fluids from the mouth and nose – once it cries, the baby can be given to the mother. Wrap the child in a dry blanket to keep warm. If the baby does not show signs of breathing or two minutes, then begin very gentle mouth-to-mouth resuscitation.

h. The placenta will usually deliver spontaneously after about ten minutes. Separation of the baby from the placenta can wait until help from the emergency services arrive.

i. Otherwise tie the umbilical cord securely with two sterile threads, one placed about 15 cm from the baby's navel, the other at about 20 cm, and the cord can be severed between the two ties with a sterile scissors or knife. Make sure that no bleeding is evident from the child's side of the cut cord.

Paediatric Emergencies

Introduction

Infants and children are also prone to accidents and emergencies, maybe more so than adults in some circumstances. While the general First Aid principles described for adults will also apply in the paediatric patient, special considerations may need to be taken into consideration when applying first aid measures.

Choking

Children, especially preschool toddlers will put most things into their mouth and risk aspirating objects into their trachea (windpipe) rather than oesophagus (food pipe). In many cases this is witnessed by parents or bystanders and the child will suddenly look distressed, begin to cough and choke.

- *Children: back blows: If* old enough, the child should be encouraged to cough. If this is ineffective, the cough is becoming less forceful and the child becomes more distressed and turns a grey-blue colour, they require assistance to help remove the foreign body. The rescuer should support the child from behind using one arm and, with the child leaning forwards, delivers 5 sharp and forceful blows using his/her free hand. These blows are administered by holding the free arm flexed at the elbow and slightly flexed at the wrist (similar to the slapping position), and delivered to the middle of the child's back in quick succession (Figure 1). The point of maximal force needs to be the heel of the hand. Sufficient and sudden force needs to be generated to create a shock wave that, hopefully, will dislodge the foreign body that is then coughed up by the child.

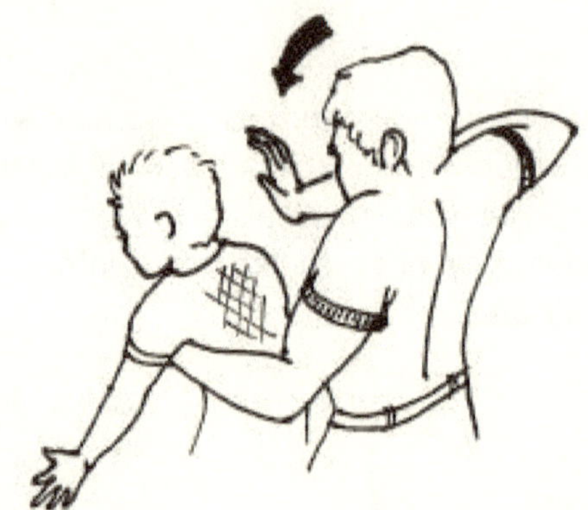

Figure 1: Delivering back blows to choking child

- *Children: abdominal thrusts:* If the five back blows are unsuccessful, the child is then turned around and administered the Heimlich manoeuvre. One hand is bunched into a fist and paced in the centre of the upper abdomen just beneath the ribcage, whist the second hand is clenched over the first. Using both arms, the rescuer administers a sudden upwards and inward jolt and repeats this 5 times (Figure 2). If still unsuccessful, these abdominal thrusts are then followed by 5 back blows and the sequence repeated until the foreign body is dislodged. If the child stops breathing and passes out, the rescuer needs to commence basic life support; if the foreign body is removed and the child recovers, he/she should be placed in the recovery position (Figure 3).

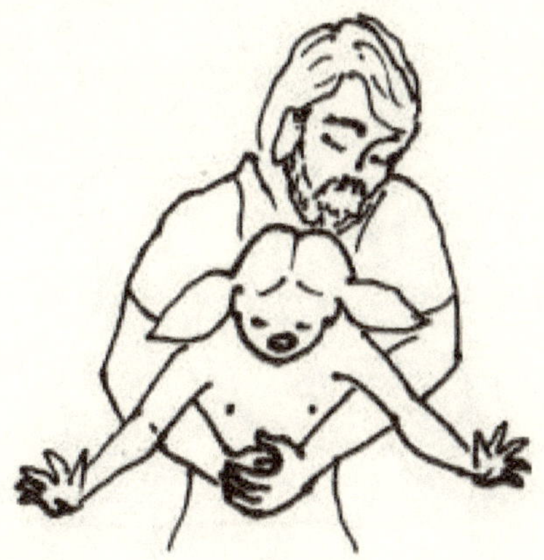

Figure 2: Delivering abdominal thrusts to choking child

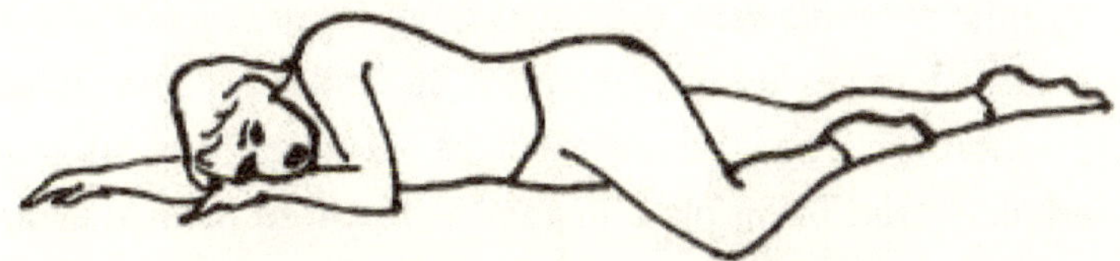

Figure 3: Recovery position for children

- *Infants: back blows:* In the case of small infants, the baby' coughing effort needs to be assessed. If this is ineffective, the cough is becoming less forceful and the infant becomes more distressed and turns a grey-blue colour, the rescuer needs to administer 5 back blows. These are similar to those administered to older children (see above) but require less force. The rescuer should be seated with the infant positioned slightly tilted downwards (sloping away from the rescuers body) and held face down on the rescuer's thighs (Figure 4).

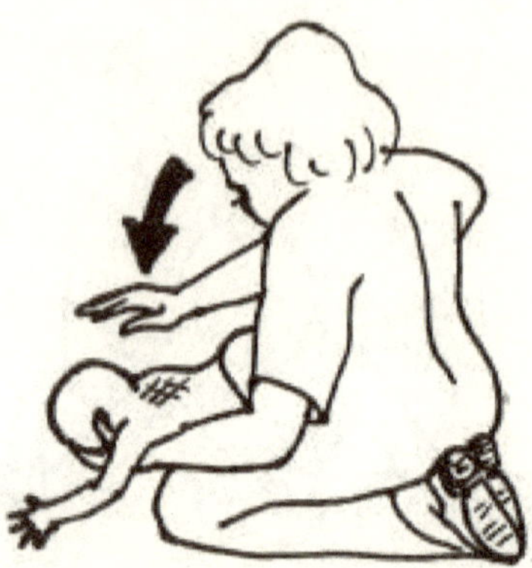

Figure 4: Delivering back blows to choking infant

- *Infants: chest blows:* If the back blows are unsuccessful, the infant is turned and held facing upwards but still in a slightly head-down position on the rescuer's thighs. 5 chest thrusts are then administered by using 2 fingers of the free hand that are kept extended and stiff and placed over the lower part of the infant's sternum (breastbone). These are then pressed onto the breastbone suddenly and with sufficient force to compress the chest and create a shock wave (Figure 5). These thrusts can then be alternated with 5 back blows, and the sequence repeated, until the foreign body is expelled.

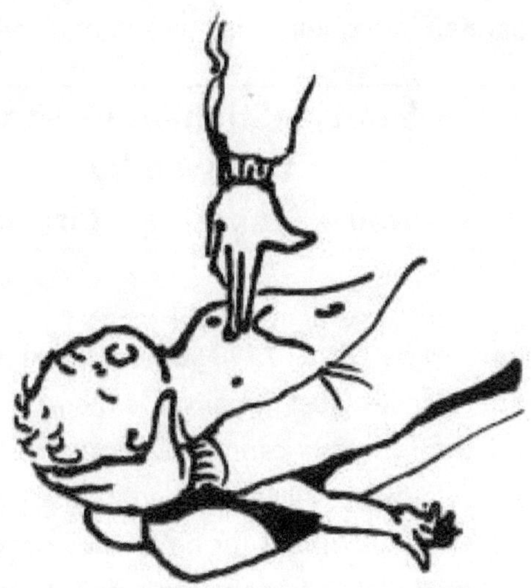

Figure 5: Delivering chest thrusts to choking infant

If the infant stops breathing and passes out, the rescuer needs to commence basic life support; if the FB is removed and the baby recovers, he/she should be placed in the recovery position.

Children and infants who stop breathing and collapse

- *The Child who stops breathing and collapses:* Children who stop breathing and collapse for whatever reason will rapidly also suffer cardiac arrest and will require 'cardiorespiratory resuscitation' (CPR). The sequence of CPR is not unlike that for adults, but with some modifications that address the fact that children initially experience respiratory rather than cardiac arrest. The process has been altered during the COVID19 pandemic.

The **pre-pandemic sequence** can be summarised as **SSS ABC**:

Safety – Stimulate – Shout
followed by
Airway – Breathing – Circulation

- *Victim known to be COVID 19 negative:* Hence, first and foremost any potential rescuer must remain **S**afe themselves and should not approach a victim if this cannot be ensured. They should then **St**imulate the victim by calling out loudly close by and, if there is no response, they should **S**hout for help. They or preferably another bystander should dial **112** and relate details to the dispatcher. The victim's **A**irway should then be assessed by opening the mouth by tilting the head slightly backwards whilst lifting the chin with the other hand. Any obvious and VISIBLE foreign body in the mouth should be removed. 'Blind' scopes in the mouth should never be attempted. Whilst getting close to the victim's face, the victim's breathing is assessed by looking, listening, and feeling for breathing movements on the rescuer's face for <u>no more than 10 seconds</u>. If not breathing, 5 rescue mouth-to-mouth breaths are delivered by the rescuer who takes in a normal breath, makes a seal over the victim's mouth, and blows in steadily (Figure 6a). If these do not result in chest movement, the mouth-to-mouth position should be adjusted, and the rescue breaths repeated. If the breaths are effective but the victim still shows no signs of life (e.g., groans, moves, starts breathing), the rescuer should administer 15 chest compressions. The heel of one hand is placed on the middle of the chest (middle of the breastbone) with the arm locked (straight) at the elbow and the shoulders positioned vertically above the point of contact. The second hand clasps the first with the fingers interlocking, again with a straight elbow and vertically above the middle of the chest (Figure 6b). Using a 'rocking' motion and the rescuer's body weight rather than direct 'pushing', the rescuer depresses the chest by about 1/3 of the front-to-back distance of the victim (several centimetres in practice) and repeats this 15 times at a rate of around 100 per minute, allowing time for the chest to re-expand after each compression. This is then followed by 2 breaths (as above) and the 15:2 sequence repeated until the victim recovers, or help arrives.

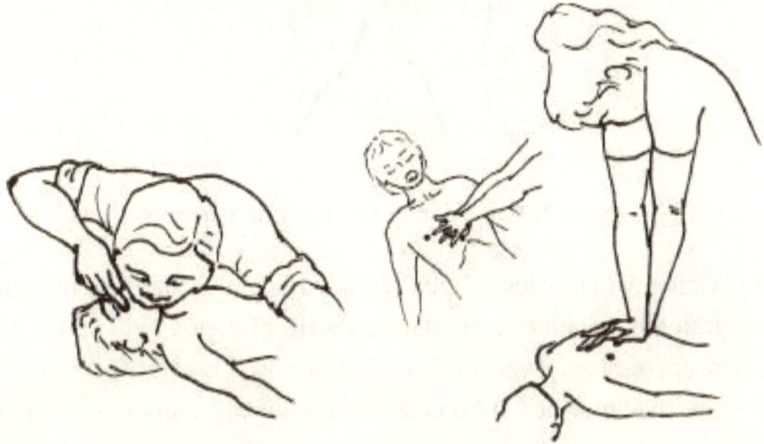

Figure 6a and 6b: Position for rescue breaths & chest compressions during CPR

In all cases, if an **Automated External Defibrillator (AED)** is available, it should be opened and attached and used as guided by the automatic voice prompts.

- *Infant who stops breathing and collapses:* The CPR sequence is similar for infants, expect that mouth-to-mouth breaths are changed for rescuer's mouth to infant's mouth and nose together. For small children, compressions may be delivered using one hand alone, in the same position as above. For infants, the hands are encircled around the chest and the midpoint of the sternum is compressed with the thumbs, again depressing the chest 1/3 of the diameter in a 15:2 ratio with rescue breaths.

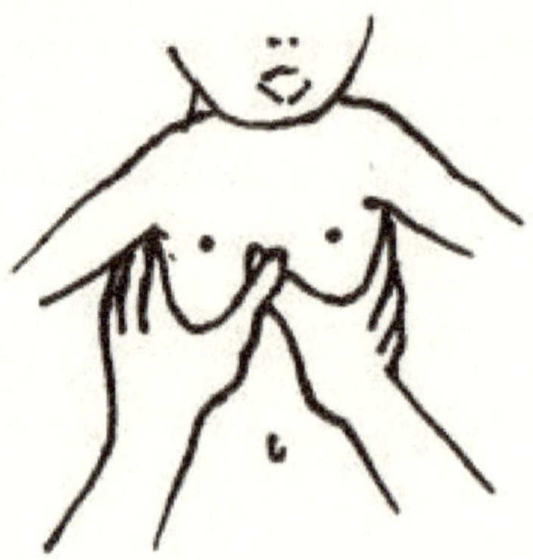

Figure 7: Two-thumb compressions in infants

- *Victim with unknown COVID 19 status:* Often collapsed children are found by relatives who may be aware of their COVID status or are prepared to deliver full CPR. If in doubt, it is safer to assume that the child may be COVID positive and the CPR sequence is modified, as follows:

The initial safe approach is unchanged, but the rescuer should take precautions and, at the very least wear a face mask, ideally with protective apron, gloves, and face shield. The airway is opened with the head-tilt, chin-lift manoeuvre but signs of breathing are looked for without getting close to the victim's face. If not breathing, the victim's nose and mouth should be covered with a cloth and compression-only CPR is delivered at a rate of around 100 per minute until the victim recovers or help arrives.

Infections and emergencies

High Fever: Most children tolerate high fevers well. Some, however, may develop complications (see below), and many conditions are exacerbated if the fever remains uncontrolled. For these reasons, fever should be managed by simple cooling and administration of paracetamol. The latter can be given by mouth or the rectal route, depending on the age, condition and cooperation of the child (see Table 1 for doses). Excessive clothing should be removed, and the child sponged gently with water at room temperature (and not immersed into cold water). Paracetamol may be repeated at intervals of six hours. Non-steroidal anti-inflammatory drugs (NSAIDS) such as ibuprofen and diclofenac can also be given, sometimes alternating with paracetamol in resistant fevers, but repeated not more than every 8 hours.

Table 1: Doses for paracetamol in children

AGE	80mg SUPPOSITORY	120mg/5ml SYRUP	125mg SUPPOSITORY
3-6 months	1	2.5 ml	1
6-24 months		5 ml	2
2-4 years		7.5 ml	
4-6 years		10 ml	

AGE	250mg/5ml SYRUP	500mg TABLETS
6-8 years	5 ml	1/2
8-10 years	7.5 ml	3/4
10-12 years	10 ml	1
12-16 years	15 ml	1 1/2

- *Croup:* This common infection is caused by respiratory viruses that result in inflammation and swelling around the upper windpipe (trachea) and voice box (larynx). Infants and young children are generally affected, and present with symptoms of a cold (snuffles, cough, often without temperature). This often progresses over a couple of days into a harsh barking cough, worse at night, sometimes associated with a crowing noise (stridor) on inhalation. Simple remedies ae often ineffective and, if the child is unduly distressed, they should be kept calm, any fever treated with paracetamol (see Table 1) and, if available, a dose of steroid (prednisolone) given. This may be administered rectally or as a syrup in a dose of around 2mg/kg body weight. Children with marked distress with breathing (making unusually strenuous efforts, those with a loud stridor, unrelenting harsh barking cough, looking tired) should be reviewed in hospital. Here, a dose dexamethasone is given with or without admission.

- *Serious infections and meningitis:* Although serious infections are now uncommon due to widespread vaccination, some children may still develop life-threatening septicaemia (infection in the blood) or meningitis (infection in the fluid that circulates within and around the brain). These children are usually very unwell, often with a high fever, extreme lethargy or unrousable, and may have severe headaches (if old enough to complain), vomiting and neck stiffness (especially on forward flexion, i.e., unable to bend their head such that their chin touches their chest). They will dislike bright light (photophobic) and loud noise. In some cases, some or all of the above may be associated with a rapidly evolving, diffuse irregular rash made up of different-sized dark red/purple patches that do not fade/disappear if pressed with a clear glass. Children presenting with these symptoms should be given paracetamol, fluids if tolerated and referred immediately to hospital.

Seizures and faints

- *Seizures with a fever:* In children usually aged between 6 months - 6 years, fevers may induce extreme shakiness (rigors or tremors), hallucinations and sometimes full-blown seizures (febrile convulsions). Although frightening, especially when occurring for the first time, these are hardly ever serious. The child will suddenly blank out, lose visual focus, stiffen, and then experience shaking of all four limbs (rhythmic jerking). They would be unresponsive at the time and, occasionally, will turn blue around the lips, with or without frothing at the mouth and/or urinary incontinence. Episodes usually last well under 5 minutes and these children then 'come-to' slowly. They should now be placed in the recovery position. Recovery followed by drowsiness and sleeping after a febrile seizure is common.

  Prevention is ideal and, for those children known to be prone to febrile seizures, their parents should treat any fever aggressively by removing excessive clothing, tepid sponging with water at room temperature and giving paracetamol by the rectal route (for dosage, see Table 1). Any objects around the mouth such as pacifiers and soothing blankets should be removed but there should be no attempt to insert one's fingers in the child's mouth. Similarly, the limbs should not be restrained and allowed to jerk.

- *Seizures without a fever:* Non febrile seizures are less common, and although most are of unknown cause (idiopathic), some may be due to underling neurological problems. The initial management for these children is the same as for febrile seizures (see above) without cooling and administration of paracetamol. Parents of children who have epilepsy and suffer with repeated seizures, will have medication that they can give by the oral (midazolam) or rectal routes (diazepam) in the event that seizures are prolonged (more 5 minutes). Children suffering these types of seizure, especially for the first time, should be reviewed by a doctor.

- *Faints:* Faints (or vasovagal episodes) are very common and result from a sudden fall in blood pressure and, therefore, circulation to the brain. They usually arise in a typical setting of a child who may not have had something to eat for a while (e.g., missed breakfast), and was standing in the heat/crowded and/or poorly ventilated room. They suddenly feel lightheaded, turn pale and slump to the floor. Some facial or limb twitching is possible but jerking, injury and incontinence are unusual and more indicative of seizures. If drowsy but conscious they should be instructed to sit and place their head down between their knees (Figure 8). The brow can be cooled with a wet facecloth, tight neckwear loosened and given a sugary drink. In addition, those children who 'pass-out' should be positioned in the supine position, and their legs raised slightly off the ground using 1-2 cushions (Figure 9). They should not be allowed to get up until feeling better without any dizziness or light-headedness.

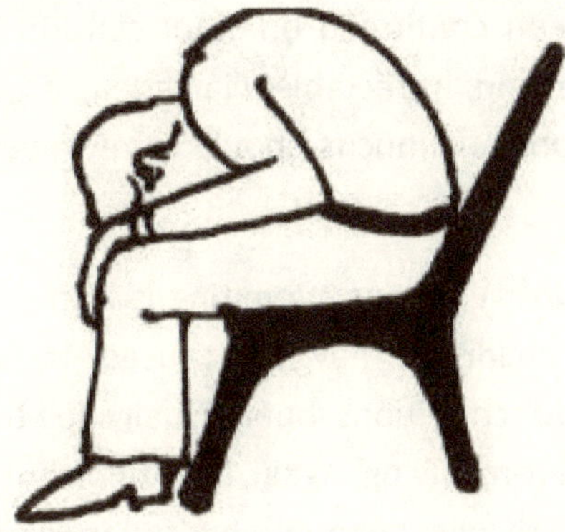

Figure 8: Head down position for child feeling faint

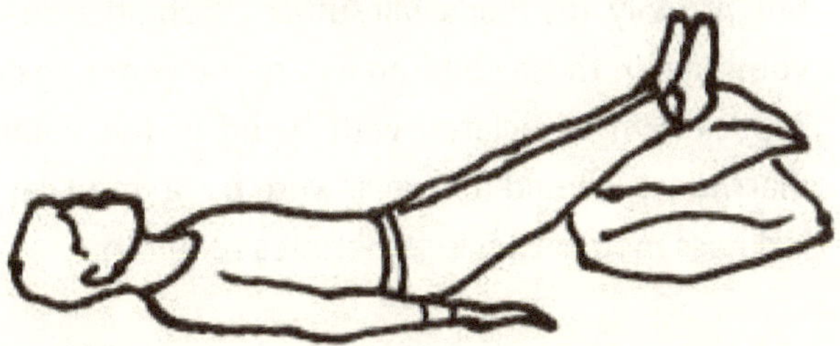

Figure 9: Supine position for child who has fainted

Diarrhoea, vomiting and dehydration

- *Intractable diarrhoea:* Diarrhoea is extremely common in young children and is usually self-resolving. The most important thing is to ensure these children receive frequent amounts of fluids. Rehydration salts bought over the counter may be used, but virtually any fluids will suffice. Dairy products may need to be omitted for a couple of these if this appears to make the diarrhoea worse. A probiotic once daily for three days will help in most cases but antibiotics should be avoided. These are only indicated with specific organisms that have been confirmed on stool culture. Those children with profuse and intractable diarrhoea, especially if associated with blood and mucus, should be reviewed by a medical team.

- *Intractable vomiting:* Vomiting is also extremely common in young children, may be caused by or associated with numerous conditions, but is usually due to minor 'gastric bugs' and is self-resolving. Again, it is important to ensure that these children receive adequate hydration, given best via small but frequent amounts of fluids. Rehydration salts may be used, but virtually any fluids will suffice. Probiotics do not help with vomiting. In those children where the vomiting doesn't settle, especially if associated with blood in the vomitus and also diarrhoea, should be reviewed by a medical team. Anti-sickness medication is sometimes required.

- *Dehydration:* Children where vomiting and diarrhoea occur together, and especially if both are profuse, run the risk of becoming dehydrated. These children may develop a fast heart and/or respiratory rate, cold and pale peripheries, sunken eyes, a dry tongue, decreased urine output and level of activity and, if severe, decreased conscious level. They should be given small but frequent amounts of fluids, paracetamol for any associated fever, and referred urgently for assessment by a medical team.

Head injury

Children, especially boisterous toddlers, are forever falling and hitting their heads. Most do not come to any harm and, after a brief cry, will recover and return to normal within a few minutes. The height of the fall or force of the impact may not be good indicators of severity. Hence, any child who has sustained a head injury and doesn't recover quickly requires medical review. The warning signs following a head injury would include children who appear drowsy, confused or disorientated, those who vomit repeatedly, and those who seem to have altered speech, gait coordination and/or eye orientation (squint). Children who seemed to have sustained a significant blow and are concussed, should be kept lying down and calm, moved as little as possible and taken or referred to hospital for review.

- *Neck injury:* In the event that a head injury may also be associated with neck injury (e.g., falls from a height, road traffic accidents, etc.), then the neck needs to be stabilised. A rescuer needs to use both hands to 'fix' the head in line with the torso and, therefore, prevent the neck from rotating in any direction (Figure 10). This position must be maintained at all times, and not interrupted until the emergency medical team take over the child's care.

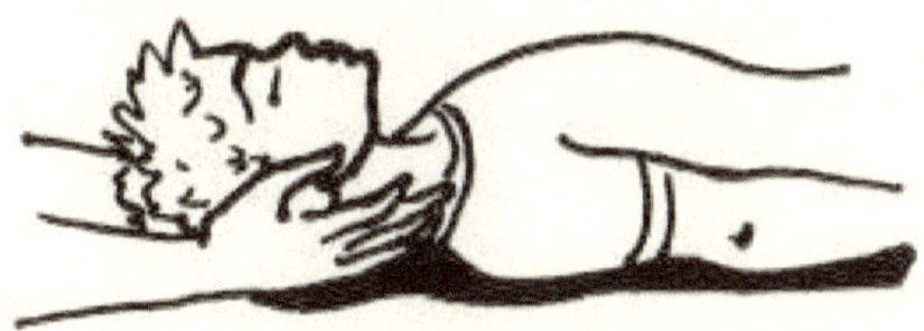

Figure 10: In-line stabilisation of the neck

Emergency Numbers

Introduction

The telephone number/s to dial in case of an emergency varies from one country to another. The generally used emergency access numbers are 112 [Europe] and 911 [U.S.A.]. These two numbers will often connect one to an emergency dispatch office. [1]

North America

- In the North American continent, the U.S.A., Canada, Bermuda, and Mexico: **911** is the emergency number which will connect you to all the emergency services – police, ambulance, fire brigade.
- The exception includes the French Territory: Saint Pierre and Miquelon where the emergency services number is 112.

Central America

- This region, in general, has yet to adopt a universal emergency number.

Country	Police	Ambulance	Fire
Clipperton Island		112	
Belize **Costa Rica** **Panama**		911	
Guatemala	110	128	122
El Salvador	911	132	913
Honduras	911	195	198
Nicaragua	118	128	115

---

[1] https://en.wikipedia.org/wiki/List_of_emergency_telephone_numbers

Caribbean and South America

- The region has generally adopted the **911** standard emergency number for all services. The McMurdo Station in Antarctica similarly uses the 911 emergency number.
- Exceptions include:

Country	Police	Ambulance	Fire
Guadeloupe Martinique Falkland Islands French Guiana		112	
Dominica Guyana South Georgia South Sandwich Islands		999	
Colombia		123	
Suriname		115	
Cuba	106	104	105
Curacao	911	912	911
Haiti	114	116	115
Trinidad and Tobago	911	811	990
Jamaica	119	110	
Brazil	190	192	193
Chile	133	131	132

Europe

- In Europe: **112** is the emergency number you can dial free of charge from fixed and mobile phones everywhere in the EU. It will get you straight through to all the emergency services – police, ambulance, fire brigade. National emergency numbers may also still in use concurrently alongside 112.
- Exceptions include the following countries:

Country	Police	Ambulance	Fire
Albania	129	127	128
Andorra	110	116	118
Austria	112	144	122
Azerbaijan	102	103	101
Belarus	102	103	101
Bosnia and Herzegovina	122	124	123
Germany	110	112	
Greece	100	166	199
Kosovo	192	194	193
Liechtenstein	117	144	118
Republic of North Macedonia	192	194	193
Monaco	17	15	18
Montenegro	122	124	123
Norway	112	113	110
San Marino	113	118	115
Serbia	112	194	193
Slovakia	158	155	150
Switzerland	117	144	118
Ukraine	102	103	101

Oceania

- This region, in general, has yet to adopt a universal emergency number. Australia adopts the **0** standard emergency number for all services.

Country	Police	Ambulance	Fire
Australia		0	
American Samoa **Fiji** **Guam** **Marshall Islands** **Micronesia** **Palau** **Solomon Islands** **Tonga** **Tuvalu**		911	
French Polynesia **New Caledonia** **Vanuatu**		112	
Cook Islands	999	998	996
Kiribati **Samoa**		999	
Nauru	110	111	112
New Zealand		111	
Papua New Guinea	112	111	110

Asia

- This region, in general, has yet to adopt a universal emergency number.

Country	Police	Ambulance	Fire
Bahrain Bangladesh Myanmar Hong Kong Qatar Macau United Arab Emirates		999	
Jordan Philippines Saudi Arabia		911	
British Indian Ocean Territory East Timor India Indonesia Iraq Kazakhstan Kuwait Tajikistan Turkmenistan		112	
Christmas Island Cocos Islands		0	
Afghanistan	119	112	119
Bhutan	113	112	110
Brunei	993	991	995
Cambodia	117	119	118
People's Republic of China	110	120	119
Iran	110	115	125
Israel	100	101	102
Japan	110	119	
Kyrgyzstan	102	103	101

Country	Police	Ambulance	Fire
Democratic People's Republic of Korea	*local numbers only*		8119
Republic of Korea	112	119	
Laos	191	195	190
Lebanon	999 or 112	140	175
Maldives	119	102	118
Malaysia	999		994
Mongolia	105		
Nepal	100	102	101
Oman	9999		
Pakistan	15	115 and 1122	16
Singapore	999	995	
Sri Lanka	119	110	
Syria	112	110	113
Republic of China (Taiwan)	110	119	
Thailand	191 or 911	1669	199
Uzbekistan	102	101	103
Vietnam	113	115	114
Yemen	194	191	

Africa

- This region, in general, has yet to adopt a universal emergency number.

Country	Police	Ambulance	Fire
Ascension Island Kenya Saint Helena Sudan [incl. Southern Region Zambia Zimbabwe]		999	
Cameroon Ghana Guinea-Bissau Mayotte Nigeria Réunion Sao Tome and Principe Seychelles		112	
Ethiopia Liberia		911	
Libya		1515	
Western Sahara		150	
Algeria	1548	14	
Angola	113	112	115
Benin Burundi	117	112	118
Botswana	999	997	998
Burkina Faso	17	112	18
Cape Verde	132	130	131
Central African Republic	117	1220	118
Chad	17	2251-4242	18
Comoros	17	772-03-73	18
Republic of Congo	117		118
Djibouti	17	19	18
Country	Police	Ambulance	Fire

Egypt	122	123	180
Equatorial Guinea	114	115	112
Eritrea	113	114	116
Gabon	1730	1300	18
Gambia	117	116	118
Guinea	117	18	442-020
Ivory Coast	110	185	180
Lesotho	123	121	122
Madagascar	117	124	118
Malawi	997	998	999
Mali	17	15	18
Mauritius	112	114	115
Mauritania	117	101	118
Morocco	19	15	
Mozambique	119	117	198
Namibia	10 111	depending on town/city	
Niger	17	15	18
Rwanda	112	912	112
Senegal	17	18	1515
Sierra Leone	19	999	
Somalia	888	999	555
South Africa	10 111	10 177	
Swaziland	999	977	933
Tanzania	112	114	115
Togo	117	8200	118
Tristan da Cunha	999	911	999
Tunisia	197	190	198
Uganda	112	911	112

Contributors

This work is the result of a multi-contributor effort by professionals in various fields of emergency and general medicine. Their sterling contribution is acknowledged. Contributors included:

- Dr Luke Abela – Medical doctor working in the Department of of Orthopaedics, Trauma and Sports Medicine, Mater Dei Hospital, Malta.
- Prof Simon Attard Montalto – Consultant Paediatrician, University Hospital of Malta and Head of the Paediatric Department within the Faculty of Medicine & Surgery of the University of Malta.
- Dr Sarah Cuschieri – Physician in Endocrinology and Public Health, University Hospital of Malta and Lecturer within the Faculty of Medicine & Surgery of the University of Malta; Member of the Grand Priory of the Maltese Islands – MHOSLJ.
- Dr Joseph Debono – Consultant in Surgery, University Hospital of Malta and Senior Lecturer within the Faculty of Medicine & Surgery of the University of Malta; Hospitaller of the Grand Priory of the Maltese Islands – MHOSLJ.
- Dr Raymond Gatt – Consultant Orthopaedic Surgeon, University Hospital of Malta and Senior Lecturer within the Faculty of Medicine & Surgery of the University of Malta; Council Member of the Grand Priory of the Maltese Islands – MHOSLJ.
- Dr Jonathan Joslin – Consultant in Emergency Medicine, University Hospital of Malta and Senior Lecturer within the Faculty of Medicine & Surgery of the University of Malta.
- Martin Käser DEBS – Rescue Service Paramedic and Aqua Med Helpline (travel & diving medicine) Medical Instructor in Germany and Tennessee, U.S.A.; Head of Khäser zu Raab Institute Heilbronn, Germany; Commander Emeritus of the Württemberg Commandery of the Grand Bailiwick of Germany – MHOSLJ.

- Dr Kim Sammut MD, MRCS – Medical doctor and specialist trainee in Orthopaedics, Trauma and Sports Medicine, Mater Dei University Hospital, Malta.
- Prof Charles Savona-Ventura – Consultant Obstetrician-Gynaecologist (retired), University Hospital of Malta and Head of the Obstetrics-Gynaecology Department within the Faculty of Medicine & Surgery of the University of Malta, University of Malta; International Grand Hospitaller & Grand Prior of the Maltese Islands – MHOSLJ.
- Dr Christine Vella – Medical doctor working in the Department of of Orthopaedics, Trauma and Sports Medicine, Mater Dei Hospital, Malta.

www.ingramcontent.com/pod-product-compliance
Lightning Source LLC
Chambersburg PA
CBHW051454250726
48655CB00001B/403